EARLY DIAGNOSIS AND PREVENTION OF GENETIC DISEASES

BOERHAAVE SERIES
FOR POSTGRADUATE
MEDICAL EDUCATION
Nr. 11

PROCEEDINGS OF BOERHAAVE COURSES
ORGANIZED BY
THE FACULTY OF MEDICINE, UNIVERSITY OF LEIDEN
THE NETHERLANDS

EARLY DIAGNOSIS
AND PREVENTION
OF GENETIC DISEASES

EDITED BY

L. N. WENT, D.SC., CHR. VERMEIJ-KEERS, M.D., AND
A. G. J. M. VAN DER LINDEN, PH.D.

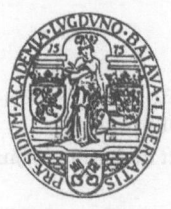

1975
LEIDEN UNIVERSITY PRESS

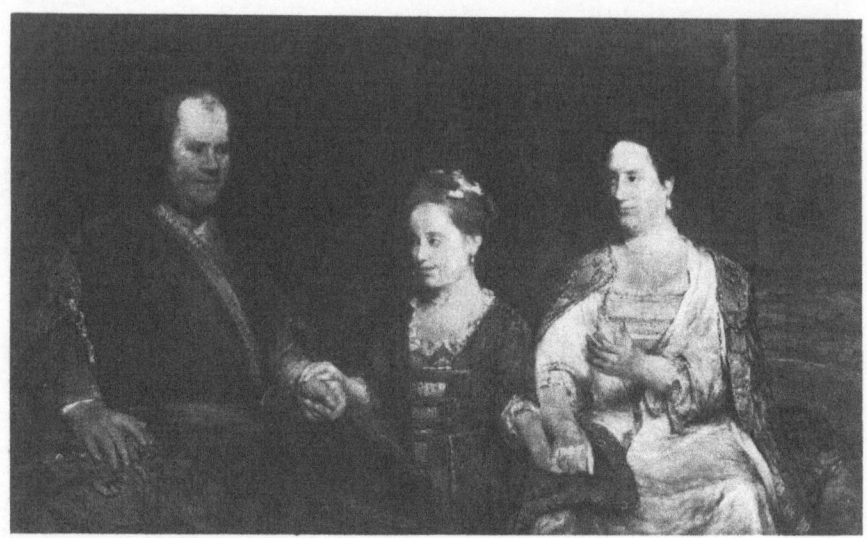

Boerhaave Family.
(Aert de Gelder, about 1723; Rijksmuseum, Amsterdam).

ISBN-13:978-94-010-1932-3   e-ISBN-13:978-94-010-1930-9
DOI: 10.1007/978-94-010-1930-9
Jacket design: E. Wijnans

© 1975 Leiden University Press, Leiden, The Netherlands
Softcover reprint of the hardcover 1st edition 1975

PREFACE

The present volume of the Boerhaave series intends to be a reflexion of our present knowledge in the expanding field of early diagnosis and prevention of inherited disorders.

Early diagnosis can mean detection of a carrier state in one or both potential parents, detection of a specific inherited disease in a previously born child or during a pregnancy at risk, or during various stages of the life of an already born individual.

The first chapters will discuss inherited disorders manifesting later in life. In Huntington's Chorea detection may be possible from the age of 20 or 30 onwards, while in myotonic dystrophy it will be seen that detection may be possible soon after birth.

Retinoblastoma serves as example of a disease manifesting in early infancy and which is partially treatable by surgical intervention. The same early onset does occur in phenylketonuria and cystic fibrosis. Both diseases provide examples of the possibilities of population screening, while in phenylketonuria an eminently succesful treatment is found in a restricted diet.

For the usually early manifesting sphingolipidoses no treatment exists as yet, but enzyme treatment might in the near future become a reality.

Spina bifida and anencephaly are not simple inherited Mendelian disorders but they are discussed in this volume because prevention is possible by antenatal diagnosis and subsequent interruption of the pregnancy if requested by the future parents. Further views on antenatal diagnosis notably in inborn errors of metabolism are presented in a following chapter.

Haemophilia is discussed as an example of a sex-linked disorder in which detection of heterozygote females is feasible in many instances.

In an overall picture of the problems and possibilities around family detection of inherited diseases some of the aspects mentioned in preceding chapters are summarised.

The difficulties and future prospects of genetic counseling and screening at the population level receive ample attention and are discussed in the second part of the book.

The last part is dedicated to ethics. It begins with explanations by the ethicists how one arrives at moral decisions and who is involved in reaching these decisions; this is followed by a general discussion.

The editors

CONTENTS

CONTRIBUTORS

G. J. P. A. ANDERS, Department of Human Genetics, University of Groningen, Groningen, The Netherlands.

TH. C. J. BEEMER, Institute of Theology, Catholic University of Nijmegen, Nijmegen, The Netherlands.

H. F. M. BUSCH, Department of Neurology, University Hospital Dijkzigt, Rotterdam, The Netherlands.

W. M. J. VAN DUYNE, Ministry of Public Health, Leidschendam, The Netherlands.

J. H. EDWARDS, Department of Human Genetics, Infant Development Unit, Birmingham, United Kingdom.

C. J. EPSTEIN, San Francisco Medical Center, University of California, San Francisco (Cal.), U.S.A.

A. DE FROE, Department of Human Genetics and Human Biology, University of Amsterdam, Amsterdam, The Netherlands.

H. GALJAARD, Department of Cellbiology, Faculty of Medicine, Erasmus University, Rotterdam, The Netherlands.

H. J. HEERING, Institute of Theology, University of Leiden, Leiden, The Netherlands.

L. P. TEN KATE, Department of Human Genetics, University of Groningen, Groningen, The Netherlands.

A. G. MOTULSKY, Division of Medical Genetics, University of Washington, Seattle (Wash.), U.S.A.

P. J. ROSCAM ABBING, Institute of Theology, University of Groningen, Groningen, The Netherlands.

K. E. W. P. TAN, 'Ooglijdersgasthuis', Utrecht, The Netherlands.

J. J. VELTKAMP, Department of Hematology, University Hospital, Leiden, The Netherlands.

L. N. WENT, Department of Human Genetics, University of Leiden, Leiden, The Netherlands.

INTRODUCTION

H. GALJAARD

Today, scientists are frequently challenged to justify their work. At the beginning of this meeting on prevention of genetic diseases I will therefore try to briefly outline the magnitude of the problem. In our country there are several hundred thousands of handicapped people, who ask our medical and social assistance. More than 20.000 of them spend their whole life in institutes, about 60.000 are in special schools and many tenths of thousands others need regular medical and social care. Apart from the financial costs this requires the daily efforts of over 30.000 doctors, teachers, nurses, psychologists and many others who are frequently under heavy physical and psychological stress. And in our country each year 8000-12000 new-borns are born with congenital abnormalities, part of which are of a hereditary nature.

Even more important than these figures is the personal suffering of the handicapped and/or his family. There is insecurity, inability, pain, sometimes physical and mental detoriation and early death or a prolonged handicapped life. Also many patients are confronted with the recurrence risk in subsequent pregnancies; this affects their family planning. In other instances couples do not dare to have any children at all because of a high genetic risk, whereas others have multiple abortions which might be associated with fetal abnormalities.

Both the personal and organizational problems outlined above, amply justify the work we are doing and also this course on early diagnosis and prevention of genetic diseases. We are still far from understanding all aspects of the 1000 patients with chromosomal aberrations, of the 2000 patients with hereditary diseases based on a gene mutation and of the 5000-9000 patients with disturbances in embryonic development, which are born each year in the Netherlands.

HUNTINGTON'S CHOREA*

L. N. WENT, M. VEGTER-VAN DER VLIS,
W. VOLKERS AND H. COLLEWIJN

This autosomal dominant inherited disorder can serve as an example for the large group of heredodegenerative neurological disorders, in which more or less well-defined areas of the central nervous system may be damaged. A biochemical basis for an error of metabolism has in practically none of these disorders been found as yet, while frequently the first symptoms become manifest after early childhood. Therefore it is understandable that therapy directed towards the primary, inherited defect is not possible today; consequently prenatal diagnosis cannot be considered either. Since Huntington's Chorea (HuCh) is the most frequent of these heredodegenerative disorders, an epidemiological and clinical approach of this disease may help in a search for earlier detection of these disorders. Earlier detection appears to be a prerequisite for prevention ever to become effective.

Many articles have been published on HuCh since the first comprehensive description of this disease in 1872 by George Huntington (1). The disease must have been known already before the 16th century in Europe and a drawing by P. Brueghel (fig. 1) represents some patients who might be affected by 'St. Vitus' dance, a name which has sometimes, probably erroneously, been used as a synonym for HuCh. Good review articles on HuCh have been written by Myrianthopoulos (2) and by Bruyn (3) while a centennial bibliography with 1963 titles has appeared in 1974 (4). Notwithstanding the considerable efforts made in the study of this disease the hundreds of patients with HuCh living in the Netherlands and the multiples of thousand living all over the Western world stand witness for our failure materially to reduce their numbers by preventive measures.

The present gene frequency of the HuCh gene in NW Europe and the U.S. might be somewhere in the order of 0.00005 to 0.0001. Consequently the frequency of gene carriers in the population (gene carriers are heterozygotes and therefore have one normal and one abnormal gene) is twice this value, around 0.0001 to 0.0002 (5). This means that of every 10.000 people between

* This work was supported by the 'Praeventiefonds'.

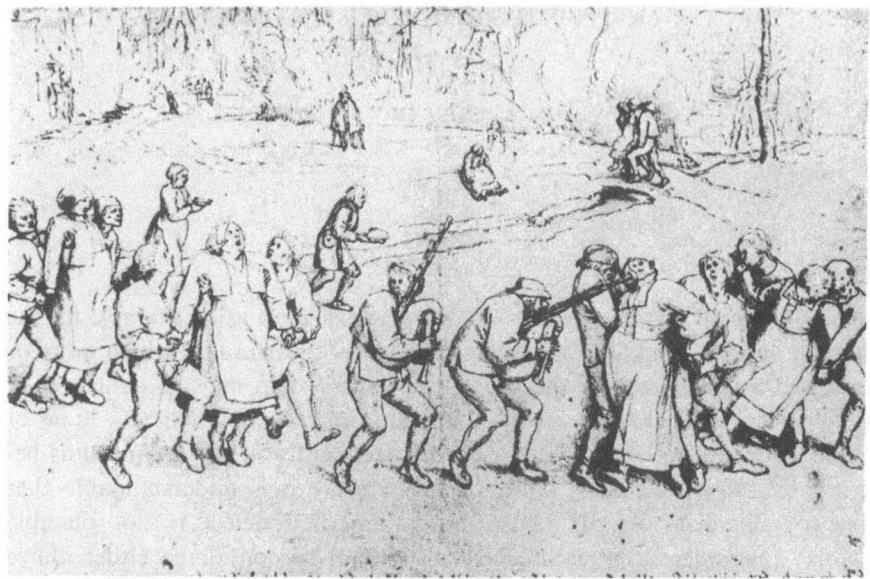

Fig. 1. Drawing by P. Brueghel the older, probably after a lost painting. (1569 A.D., courtesy Prentenkabinet-nr. 16859-Rijksmuseum, Amsterdam). Another identical drawing is in the Albertina collection, Vienna (nr. 42435).

one and two will carry the gene and be prone ultimately to develop the disease.

The most prominent, albeit not always obligate, characters of HuCh are the uncoordinated, uncontrolled choreatic movements – which may effect any part of the body but are notably visible in the extremities and the face –, disturbances of speech and the slowly progressive dementia. The disease is dramatic in its consequences specifically because its late age of onset and very slow progression. Although the peak of the apparent age of onset is around 41 years (fig. 2) the curve has a very wide spread; it has a practically identical shape to the age of death curve (fig. 2). The average overall duration of the disease calculated from these data is 14 years, but undoubtedly early symptoms of the disease have been present in many patients well before the indicated age of onset. Our own studies strongly suggest that by careful observation of persons at risk it is possible to detect the presence of the disease at least 5 to 10 years before it is recognized by the family or the patient him-(or her-)self.

In view of the wide variability of the ages at which the disease first manifests itself and of the ages at death (fig. 2) it is necessary to know whether

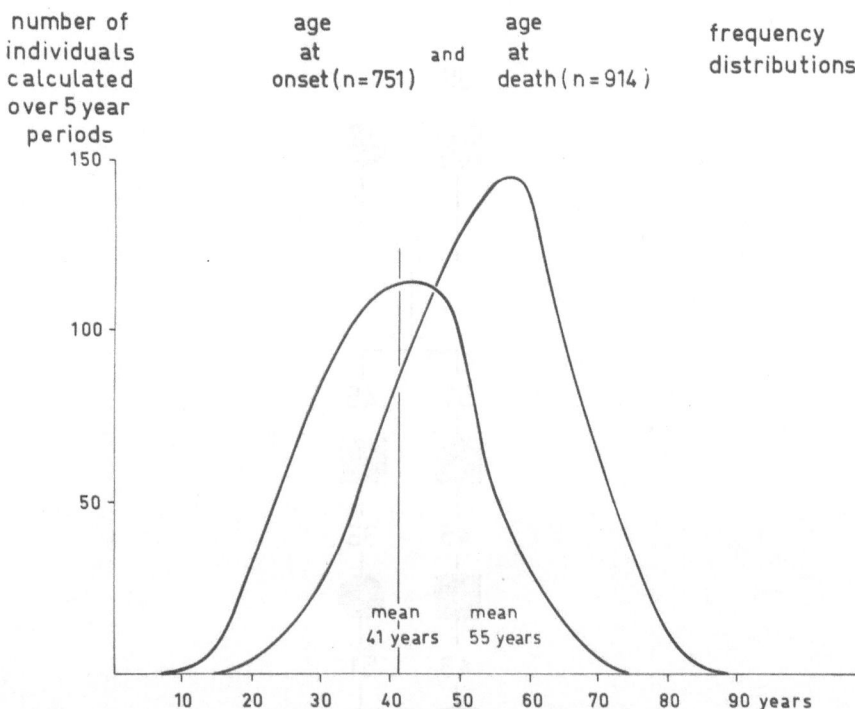

Fig. 2. Age at onset and age at death curves for combined data of 1327 patients with Huntington's Chorea in 164 pedigrees obtained from Eastern Belgium, North Western France and Holland; from a publication of Husquinet et al. (6).

these variations are genetically or environmentally determined. For this purpose two large families from the surroundings of Leiden, who do not seem to be related, were studied in greater detail (figs. 3 and 4). Family A was not included in the original study (6), family B only partially. They both belong to a low normal socio-economic class of the society with closely comparable standards of living. From these pedigrees and from the frequency distribution of their ages at onset and ages of death (figs. 5a and 5b) it is very evident (Table 1) that there must be genetic heterogeneity to explain the statistically extremely significant age differences between the two families. Notwithstanding this conclusion about the existence of different genes for Huntington's Chorea, genes which may well be alleles, there should be no doubt that also nongenetic factors play an important role in the expression of the gene(s) for HuCh. The ages at which the patients have died from the disease vary between 13 and 66 for family A and between

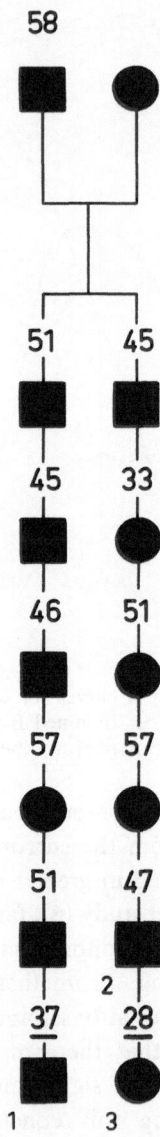

Fig. 3. Very much abbreviated pedigree of a large family (A) with Huntington's Chorea with a rather low average age at death. The ages at death are indicated for every person; if the patients were still living in 1974 their ages in that year are underlined. The total size of this family is approximately 100 with 45 known affected individuals.

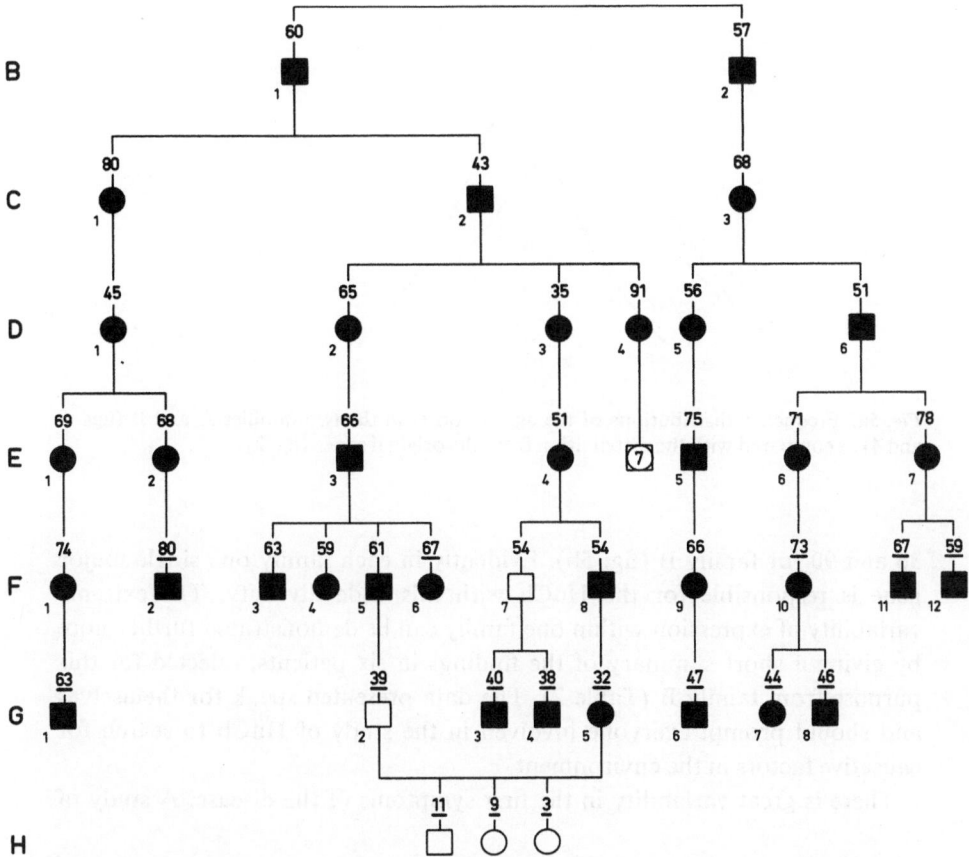

Fig. 4. Very much abbreviated pedigree of a large family (B) with a rather high average age at death. Open squares and circles indicate that the individuals were (are) not yet affected when they died, resp. in 1974. The total size of this family is approximately 400, with 90 known affected individuals.

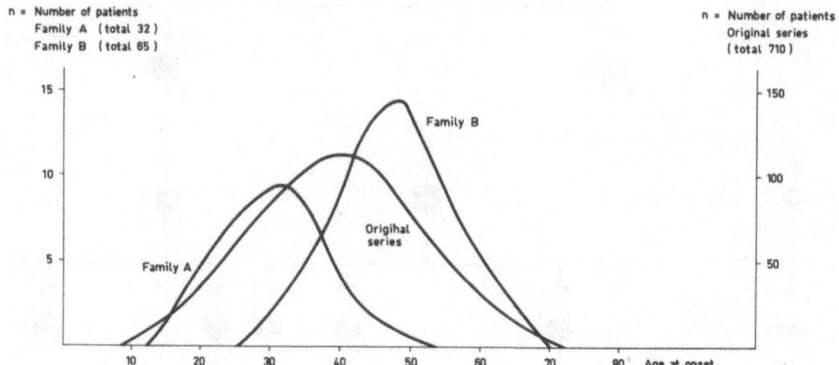

Fig. 5a. Frequency distributions of the ages at onset in the two families A and B (figs. 3 and 4) as compared with the distribution from the original series (fig. 2).

36 and 90 for family B (fig. 5b). Evidently in each family one single major gene is responsible for the HuCh with this wide diversity. The extreme variability of expression within one family can be demonstrated furthermore by giving a short summary of the findings in six patients, selected for this purpose from family B (Table 2). The data presented speak for themselves and should prompt everyone involved in the study of HuCh to search for causative factors in the environment.

There is great variability in the first symptoms of the disease. A study of

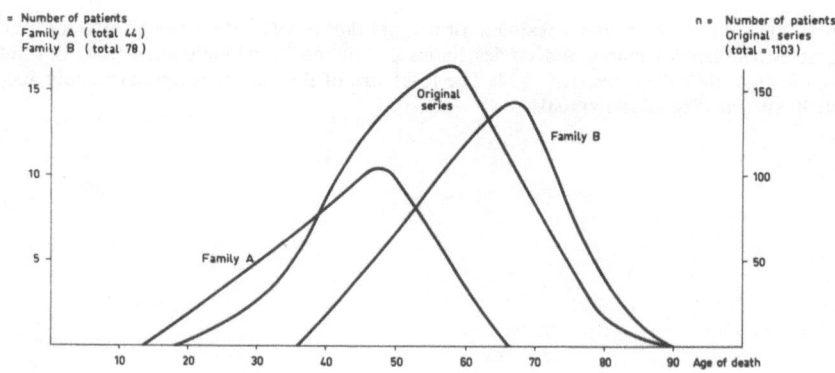

Fig. 5b. Frequency distributions of the ages of death in the same three groups.

Table 1. Mean ages at onset and mean ages of death (in years) in the two families A and B (figs. 3 and 4) and in the original series (fig. 2) excluding families A and B. The value p indicates the one sided tail probability that the age differences between families A and B are due to chance.

	AGE AT ONSET		AGE OF DEATH	
Family A	32.5 (n = 32)		47.1 (n = 44)	
		$p = 10^{-10}$		$p = 10^{-12}$
Family B	47.4 (n = 65)		63.9 (n = 78)	
Remainder	40.6 (n = 710)		54.9 (n = 1103)	

Table 2. A summary of the salient clinical features of patients with HuCh from family B. The first presenting symptom of the disease in each patient is indicated in brackets.

Patient F-2	Patient F-7	Patient G-1
onset: 60; age (1974): 80 (movements)	Death: 54 (cerebral tumour)	onset: 48; age (1974): 65 (behaviour) Psychiatric hospital: 59
movements +	No symptoms of HuCh	movements + +
rigidity —	before death	rigidity —
behaviour —		behaviour + +
dementia —		dementia + +
reflexes normal		reflexes ↗ ↗
remark: speech and writing good		

Patient G-3	Patient G-4	Patient G-7
onset: 38; age (1974): 40 (gait)	onset: 25; age (1974): 38 (movements) Psychiatric Hospital: 30 (completely rigid with contractions)	onset: 45; age (1974): 46 ('nervousness')
movements +	movements ±	movements +
rigidity —	rigidity + +	rigidity —
behaviour ±	behaviour + +	behaviour —
dementia —	dementia + +	dementia —
reflexes ↗	reflexes ↗ ↗	reflexes ↗

Table 3. A listing of some of the most prominent early signs and symptoms of Huntington's Chorea in 100 patients, from data published by Oliver (7). Usually more than one symptom has been reported in an individual patient.

Neurological		Psychiatric	
Movements	25	Anxiety	13
Gait	11	Depression	15
Speech	14	Apathy	7
	50	Tiredness, insomnia	9
Social		Suicidal attempts	4
		Emotional instability	19
Antisocial behaviour	13	Schizofreniform behaviour	12
Aberrant sexual behaviour	6	Beginning dementia	15
Persistently out of work	11		
	30		94

such symptoms (Table 3) clearly reveals that personality changes are very frequent and thus it is not only the patient wo will suffer but also his or her family. Frequently the disruption of normal family life is a consequence of

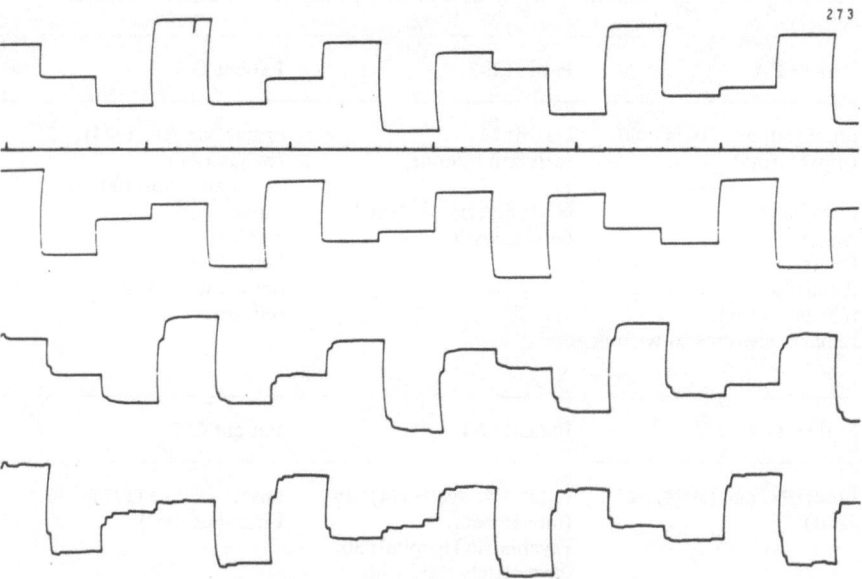

273

Fig. 6. Tracing of interrupted movements of a light spot on a screen two meters in front of the observer. The top two tracings are the horizontal and vertical components of the actual movements of the light spot, the lower two tracings are the horizontal and vertical components of the pursuit movements of the eye. The time scale between the two tracings on the top is in seconds.

a. A normal, healthy man, age 28. Normal saccadic movements.

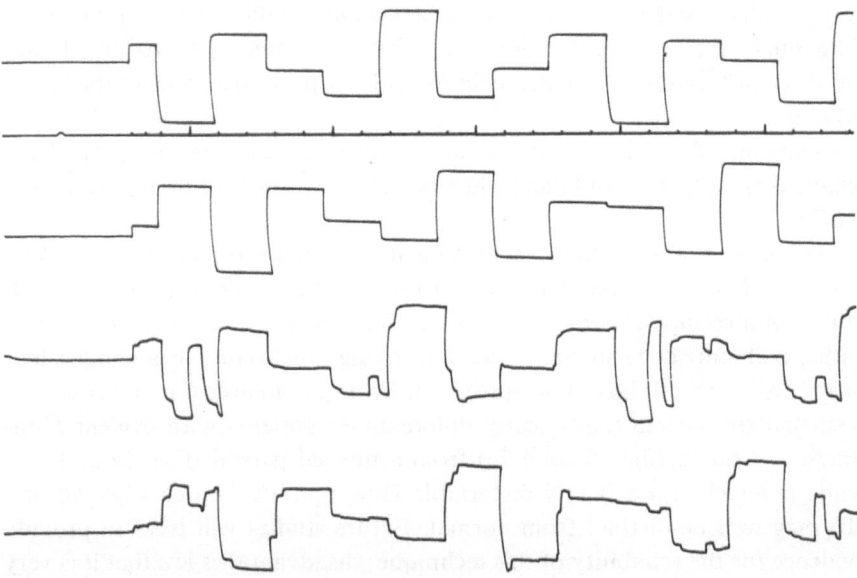

Fig. 6b. Female, age 37, with early HuCh unknown to herself.

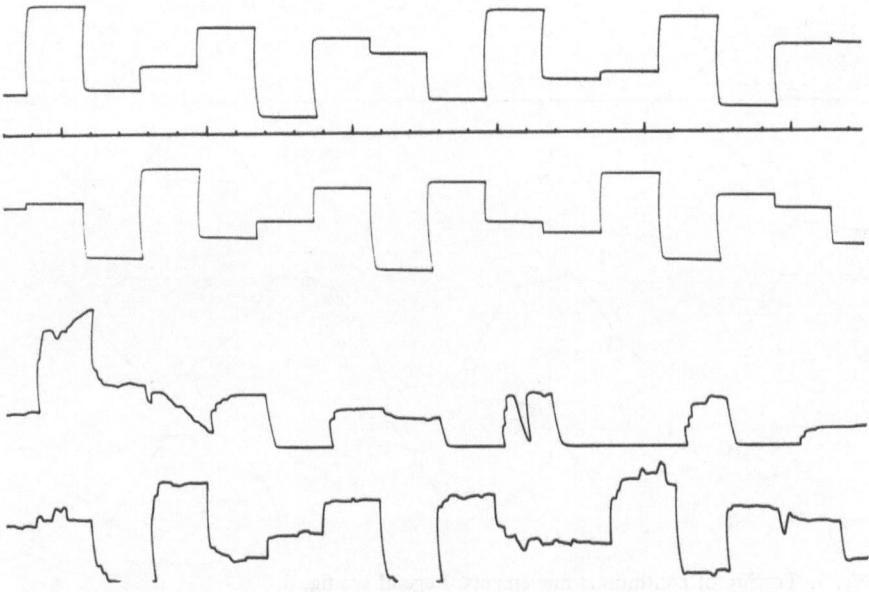

Fig. 6c. Male, age 40, with HuCh; onset at age 38 (G-3, family B).

such changes and can therefore affect a considerably greater number of individuals than the approximately one gene carrier per 10.000. Better guidance of families at risk can help to avoid or postpone some of the harmful effects.

Detection of the disease at a younger age seems an essential part of the results that have to be obtained when one wants to advance in understanding HuCh.

The method of recording eye movements, which has been discussed before (8) seemed to be a potentially useful tool for earlier detection. The availability of a set-up (9) making use of an electromagnetic induction principle with a coil embedded in a silicone rubber ring functioning as a contact lens prompted us to establish a testprogram. From the figures 6 and 7 it can be seen that the system used clearly differentiates patients with evident Huntington's Chorea (figs. 6c and 7c) from a normal person (figs. 6a and 7a), while patients with a barely discernible Huntington's Chorea (figs. 6b and 7b) may well be distinct from normal. Future studies will have to provide evidence for the reliability of this technique; disadvantages are that it is very

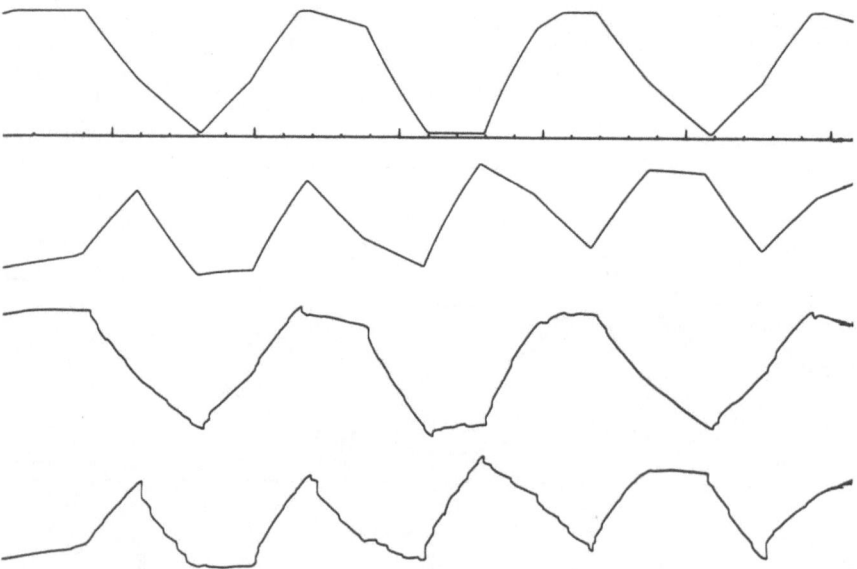

Fig. 7. Tracing of continuous movements. Legend see fig. 6.
a. A normal, healthy man, age 28. Normal saccadic movements, more evident in the vertical component.

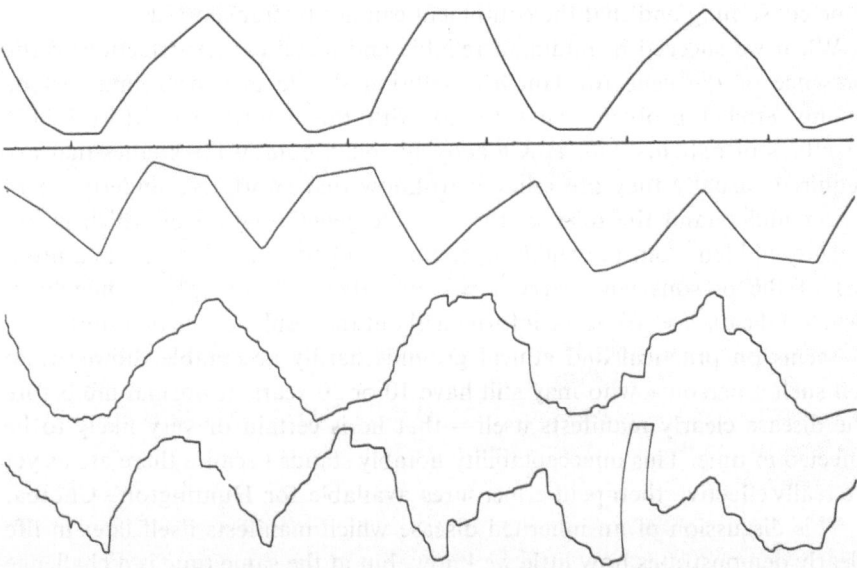

Fig. 7b. Male, age 37, with mild choreatic movements since one year (patient 1, family A).

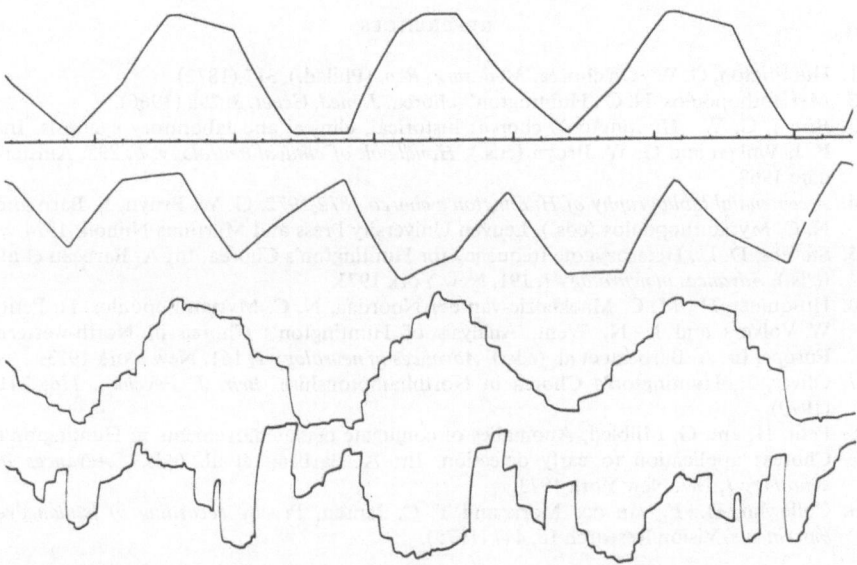

Fig. 7c. Male, age 47; onset of HuCh at least 9 years earlier; vertical component more evidently involved (G-6, family B).

time consuming and that the equipment can not be transported.

When we succeed in finding a reliable and much earlier detection of the presence of the gene for HuCh a solution should also be found for the mainly ethical problem what to do with this knowledge. Most family members of patients with HuCh actively collaborate in the studies that are required; usually they are relieved to know that efforts are undertaken to better understand the disease, the possible genetic nature of which is frequently hidden from the children, spouses and surroundings. Quite a number of the persons who carry a risk of eithei 50% or 25% ultimately to develop the disease ask to be informed about the results of the investigations. It seems on practical and ethical grounds hardly acceptable, however, to tell such a person – who may still have 10 or 20 years of normal life before the disease clearly manifests itself – that he is certain or very likely to be affected in time. This unacceptability notably stands because there are as yet no really effective therapeutic measures available for Huntington's Chorea.

This discussion of an inherited disease which manifests itself later in life clearly demonstrates how little we know, but at the same time is a challenge relentlessly to pursue the work so that many thousands of future victims may benefit from it.

REFERENCES

1. Huntington, G. W., On chorea. *Med. surg. Rep.* (Philad.), 317 (1872).
2. Myrianthopoulos, N. C., Huntington's chorea. *J. med. Genet. 3*, 298 (1966).
3. Bruyn, G. W., Huntington's chorea: historical, clinical and laboratory synopsis. In: P. J. Vinken and G. W. Bruyn (eds.), *Handbook of clinical neurology*, 6, 298. Amsterdam 1968.
4. *A centennial bibliography of Huntington's chorea 1872-1972*. G. W. Bruyn, F. Baro and N. C. Myrianthopoulos (eds.). Leuven University Press and Martinus Nijhoff, 1974.
5. Stevens, D. L., Heterozygote frequency for Huntington's Chorea. In: A. Barbeau et al. (eds.), *Advances in neurology 1*, 191. New York 1973.
6. Husquinet, H., M. C. Mackenzie-van der Noordaa, N. C. Myrianthopoulos, H. Petit, W. Volkers and L. N. Went, Analysis of Huntington's Chorea in North-western Europe. In: A. Barbeau et al. (eds.), *Advances in neurology 1*, 161. New York 1973.
7. Oliver, J., Huntington's Chorea in Northhamptonshire. *Brit. J. Psychiat. 116*, 241 (1970).
8. Petit, H. and G. Milbled, Anomalies of conjugate ocular movements in Huntington's Chorea: application to early detection. In: A. Barbeau et al. (eds.), *Advances in neurology 1*, 287. New York 1973.
9. Collewijn, H., F. van der Mark and T. C. Jansen, *Precise recording of human eye movements*. Vision Research 15, 447 (1975).

DISCUSSION

PAPER OF L.N. WENT C.S.

Delleman: Dr. Went mentioned the possibility of genetic heterogeneity; is this based exclusively on the age at onset and age of death?

Went: Yes. Due to the amount of clinical variation, it is not possible at present to distinguish different genes for Huntington's chorea properly, although I am convinced of their presence. The eye-movement test is not yet adequate but could be of help in the future.

DYSTROPHIA MYOTONICA

H. F. M. BUSCH AND C. J. HÖWELER

Dystrophia myotonica is thought to be transmitted as a monogenic auto-somal dominant trait and the risk of the disease in an offspring of a patient is 1 in 2. If fully developed, this disease is seriously incapacitating. It affects many systems besides the skeletal muscles and leads to death before the normal age, usually as a result of cardiorespiratory complications. There is, however, a great variation in expressivity. Some affected relatives may lead a normal professional life with only minor symptoms, which may be minimal or not even be known to themselves. Others may present with very early or congenital onset, often associated with mental retardation (1,2). Genetic advice, if requested at all, will be asked in general by parents or sibs of those patients who show congenital or early onset, or rapid progression of symptoms, appearing in the second decade. The main problems in genetic counseling are that a consultant may carry the gene without showing symptoms and the great variability in age of onset and progression of the disease.

The diagnosis is based upon three cardinal signs: the presence of myotonia, in addition to muscle weakness and, or, specific cataracts on slit lamp examination. Myotonia is characterized by a delayed relaxation of the muscles following contraction. In dystrophia myotonica this 'stiffness', especially of the hand muscles is rarely severe. In patients showing no myotonia on physical examination, typical myotonic discharges may be found in the electromyogram. Muscle weakness and atrophy account for a dull and expressionless face and a nasal, monotonous speech readily suggesting the diagnosis. In the arms and the legs weakness and atrophy primarily affect the distal parts. The specific cataract consists of white and coloured opacities in the anterior and posterior cortex of the lens. Additional well-recognized manifestations of the disease include cardiac abnormalities, pulmonary insufficiency, hypomotility of the gastro-intestinal tract, endocrine (hypogonadism) and mental disturbances. If such features are presenting complaints in patients, only showing slight myotonia and muscle weakness, the diagnosis of dystrophia myotonica is likely to remain obscure.

The congenital occurrence of dystrophia myotonica has recently received much interest (3,4). The main clinical features are: arthrogryposis, facial diplegia, poor sucking, respiratory insufficiency and ultimately, if these children survive, mental slowness and deficiency. The absence of myotonia and cataracts may account for the fact that this syndrome was first described more than 50 years after the original description of the disease in adults by Steinert.

Genetic counseling appears to be particularly important in congenital dystrophia myotonica. However, since the clinical picture is rather non-specific, a correct diagnosis is often not made. For some as yet unknown reason, the syndrome appears to occur only in the offspring of affected mothers. Therefore by clinical examination of the mother, supplemented by electromyography and slit lamp examination, if necessary, the true nature of the syndrome may be recognized in the child and sometimes allows an early diagnosis in the mother as well (4).

As indicated by several recent studies (5-7) on early detection of the disease, clinical examination by an experienced physician, electromyography and slit lamp examination appear to be the most reliable methods. An investigation using these methods in two large families, residing in the Rotterdam area, was prompted by a request for genetic advice from relatives. In these two families 53 relatives in 21 sibships could be examined. All together 33 patients were identified. In 20 patients the condition had not been recognized previously. In accordance with the literature clinical examination proved to be the most successful procedure since diagnostic signs were found in 26 patients. Two patients were identified by myotonic discharges in the electromyogram, three patients by slit lamp examination and one by the combination of these two methods.

Condensed pedigrees of the families are presented in figures 1 and 2.

CASE HISTORIES

Family A (fig. 1)

I 1. Died at 78 yr. Reported to have had cataracts.

II 1-4. Ages: 79, 71, 68, died at 64 yr. The patients had normal intelligence and normal professional careers. They all had specific cataracts. II 1 and 4 had had cataracts removed. In both cardiac arrest had followed general anesthesia, causing death in II 4. The living patients showed slight to moderate myotonia of the hands. Moderate muscle weakness only in II 2.

III 1. 47 yr. Single. Completed military service. Since the age of 25 stiffness of hands. Myotonia, moderate weakness and atrophy in the face, arms and legs, specific cataracts, testicular atrophy.

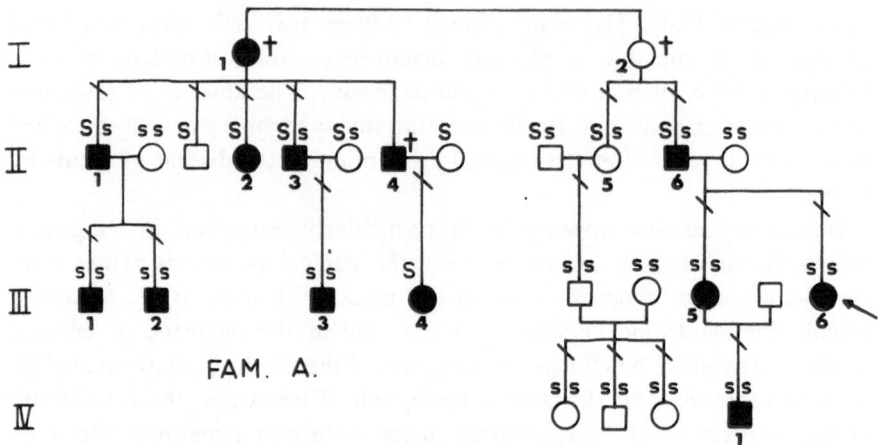

Fig. 1. Pedigree of family A. S: secretor, genotype not known. Ss: heterozygous secretor (Sese). ss non-secretor (sese). Open squares and circles indicate the individuals who are not (yet) affected in 1974. The index case is indicated by an arrow.

III 2. 41 yr. Single. Discharged from the army after 1½ yr. of service. Onset of muscular symptoms at 20 yr. Clinical picture similar to that of his brother.

III 3. 28 yr. Single. Refused for the army. Onset in second decade. Intelligence subnormal. Myotonia, slight to moderate weakness in face and hands, specific cataracts, testicular atrophy.

III 4. 16 yr. Normal neonatal period. Intelligence subnormal. Muscular symptoms since 8th yr. Myotonia, weakness of facial muscles, dysarthria, specific cataracts, atrial fibrillation.

I 2. Died at age 76 yr. No medical records available. Had walking difficulties in the last years of his life ascribed to coxarthrosis.

II 6. 66 yr. Normal professional career. Physical examination normal. Specific findings in EMG and slit lamp examination.

III 5. 38 yr. Onset of muscular symptoms at age 28 yr. Myotonia, light to moderate weakness of facial and hand muscles. Specific advanced cataracts.

III 6. 34 yr. Onset of muscular symptoms early in the third decade. Myotonia, moderate to severe weakness and atrophy of the muscles of the face, arms and legs. Non-specific lenticular opacities.

IV 1. 10 yr. Mental slowness, facial diplegia, dysarthria, slight weakness of hand muscles. Myotonic discharges in EMG, no lenticular abnormalities. History typical of congenital dystrophia myotonica.

Family B (fig. 2)

I 1. Died at the age of 80 yr. Reported to have had cataracts, no walking difficulties.
II 1. 70 yr. Operated for cataracts at the age of 50 yr. No myotonia or weakness.

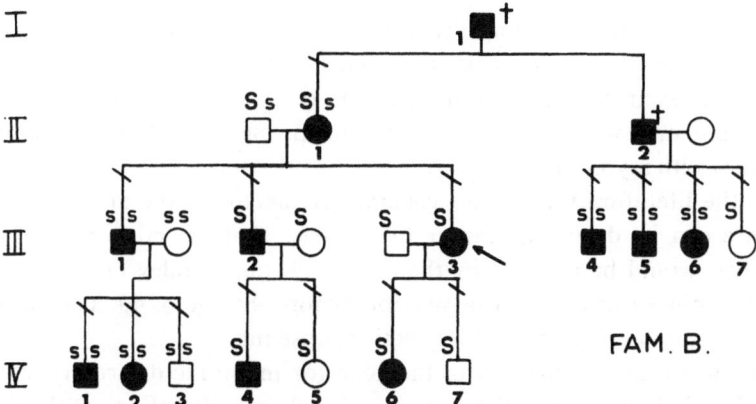

Fig. 2. Pedigree of family B. For legend see fig. 1.

Suffered three times from cardiac infarction. Atrial fibrillation. An EMG could not be performed.

III 1-3. 45, 38, 36 yr. In this kindred of five, one died at the age of 2 yr., one showed no signs of the disease. In the patients muscular symptoms appeared in the third decade, all showed the characteristic facial appearance and specific cataracts. Muscle weakness slight in III 1 and 2, moderate to severe in III 3.

IV 1. Age 20 yr. Onset not clear. Active myotonia, slight ptosis and dysarthria, non-specific lenticular changes.

IV 2. Age 10 yr. Has been hospitalized six times in the last two years because of acute gastric dilatation. Myotonic discharges in EMG. Non-specific lenticular abnormalities.

IV 3. Age 4 yr. Examination normal. Chronic obstipation and megacolon.

IV 4. Age 9 yr. Intelligence subnormal. Stiffness of the hands for a few weeks. Physical examination negative. Myotonic discharges in the EMG. Normal lenses.

IV 6. Age 13 yr. Slight retardation of motor development, following normal neonatal period. Weakness of facial muscles. Myotonic discharges in EMG. Intelligence subnormal. Normal lenses.

II 2. Died at the age of 49 yr. from pneumonia. Served as a volunteer in the army. Onset of muscular symptoms presumably in the third decade. Confined to a wheel-chair in the last years of his life.

III 4-5. Ages 25 and 24 yr. Onset of muscular symptoms at 10 yr. Myotonia, slight weakness of facial and hand muscles. Lenticular abnormalities specific in III 4, non-specific in III 5. Mental slowness.

III 6. Age 23 yr. Stiffness of the hands since 5th yr. Mental deficiency. Myotonia, non-specific lenticular abnormalities.

The findings in both families illustrate well the great variability in age of onset and severity of the disease. They also illustrate the phenomena of anticipation and progression i.e. earlier onset and increase in the severity of the condition in succeeding generations. These phenomena have been the subject of much debate in the past. Their biological significance has been denied by Penrose (8) and other authors (see 3); they are considered arte-facts. The only way definitely to settle this problem would be to study large families with myotonic dystrophy over many decades.

In the literature there is no general agreement on the age at which the disease can be detected. Harper (9) believes that detection of all affected relatives would be possible by the age of 14, but Bundey (7) states that in some families this may not be possible before the age of 40. This obviously is of paramount importance for genetic counseling.

The methods of detection of the gene for myotonic dystrophy discussed thus far all depend upon the presence of early manifestations of the disease. An indirect approach has emerged from the recognition that the gene for dystrophia myotonica is closely linked to the gene for secretor status. The practical use of this linkage in the preclinical and even antenatal detection of the gene for dystrophia myotonica has been described in detail by Schrott et al (10). For several reasons the clinical applicability of the method is very limited (6, 9, 10), but if it can be applied it is at present the only reliable way of preclinical detection of the disease.

Secretor status refers to the presence or absence in the saliva of glycoproteins with the same A, B or H specificities as the individual's blood group. It is inherited as a dominant trait, secretors either being homozygous (SeSe) or heterozygous (Sese), non-secretors being homozygous for the other allele (sese). In general, for a mating to be informative, the affected parent should be heterozygous secretor and the spouse either non-secretor or also heterozygous secretor. In addition it has to be ascertained whether the gene for dystrophia myotonica is in coupling with the secretor or non-secretor allele in the affected parent.

In family A preclinical detection by secretor status would have been possible in all patients in the third generation, with the exception of III 1 and 4. The non-secretor genotype of III 1 is the first indication in this family that the gene for dystrophia myotonica is in coupling with the non-secretor allele. The matings of II 1, 3 and 6 are informative, all non-secretors in the offspring – provided no recombi-nation occurred – will also be carrying the gene for dystrophia myotonica. Secretors in the offspring of such matings will receive the secretor allele from the affected parent and will be likely not to develop dystrophia myotonica. In a mating of the type of II 3 the 50% risk for dystrophia myotonica is reduced to 36% for secretors. In the youngest generation only III 4 might possibly have an informative secretor genotype.

In family B the secretor genotype of III 1 indicates that also in this family the gene for dystrophia myotonica is in coupling with the non-secretor allele. Both parents of IV 3 are non-secretors. Consequently, the linkage study is not helpful in the preclinical detection of the disease in this boy, suffering from megacolon, but showing no clinical signs of dystrophia myotonica. Information concerning the secretor status of the parents of III 7 could not be obtained. As a result of this practical difficulty the presence of the gene for dystrophia myotonica could not be excluded in this girl.

For several reasons family studies in dystrophia myotonica are useful. Known patients as well as those previously unidentified may benefit from succinct information to the family physician about the nature of the disorder and especially on the possible complications during general anesthesia, which may be given for cataract extraction or other operations. In addition the identification of the syndrome of congenital dystrophia myotonica will be easier and genetic counseling may more frequently be offered. At present no single satisfactory test for the preclinical detection of the gene is available. In the meantime, the knowledge of the secretor genotypes of the patients and their spouses may be of considerable help in this regard in a very limited number of cases. Finally, further insight may possibly be gained with respect to the controversial issue of the phenomena of anticipation and progression by the long term study of complete pedigrees. With respect to these phenomena dystrophia myotonica appears to be unique (3).

ACKNOWLEDGEMENTS

Dr. L. E. Nijenhuis kindly tested the secretor status. We are grateful to Mrs. J. M. Mellink-van der Hoog for secretarial assistance. This work was supported by a grant from the 'Prinses Beatrix' Fund.

REFERENCES

1. Walton, J. N., *Disorders of voluntary muscle*. Edinburgh and London 1974.
2. Zellweger, H., Myotonic dystrophy and its differential diagnosis. *Acta Neurol. Scand.* 49, suppl. 55 (1973).
3. Dyken, P. R. and P. S. Harper, Congenital dystrophia myotonica. *Neurology* (Minneapolis) 23, 465 (1973).
4. Aicardi, J., D. Conti and F. Goutières, Les formes néonatales de la dystrophie myotonique de Steinert. *J. neurol. Sci.* 22, 149 (1974).
5. Bundey, S. and C. O. Carter, Early recognition of heterozygotes for the gene for dystrophia myotonica. *J. Neurol. Neurosurg. Psychiat.* 33, 279 (1970).
6. Polgar, J. G., W. G. Bradley, A. R. M. Upton, J. Anderson, J. M. L. Howat, F. Petito, D. F. Roberts and J. Scopa, The early detection of dystrophia myotonica. *Brain 95*, 761 (1972).
7. Bundey, S., Detection of heterozygotes for myotonic dystrophy. *Clin. Genet. 5*, 107 (1974).

8. Penrose, L. S., The problem of anticipation in pedigrees of dystrophia myotonica. *Ann. Eugen. (London) 14*, 125 (1948).
9. Harper, P. S., Pre-symptomatic detection and genetic counselling in myotonic dystrophy. *Clin. Genet. 4*, 134 (1973).
10. Schrott, H. G., L. Karp and G. S. Omenn, Prenatal prediction in myotonic dystrophy: guidelines for genetic counseling. *Clin. Genet. 4*, 38 (1973).

DISCUSSION

PAPER OF H.F.M. BUSCH AND C. J. HÖWELER

Went: I was very interested to hear that congenital forms are transmitted almost exclusively through the mothers, because in Huntington's chorea there is strong evidence that the juvenile form is transmitted through an affected father!

Mrs. Mackenzie: If the father suffers from gonadal atrophy (hypogonadism) there is less chance of transmission through the father.

Busch: There is indeed a reduced fertility in males from these families, but this cannot explain why in 98% of the cases the disease is transmitted through the mother.

Motulsky: The linkage between the secretor status and myotonic dystrophy, although theoretically useful for early diagnosis of the disease, is unfortunately rarely applicable in these particular situations. Therefore, from the point of view of research strategy it has become much more important to try to find the biochemical equivalent of what the disease does, so that we can diagnose directly.

Busch: But if a woman asks advice you are compelled to investigate the secretor status, in the hope that the family is informative (a chance of 1 in 5).

RETINOBLASTOMA

K. E. W. P. TAN

Retinoblastoma is a malignant tumour originating from the retina; it is often multifocal and can affect one or both eyes. It develops in the first years of life in approximately 1 in 15,000 to 1 in 30,000 children. The affection is sometimes hereditary.

The disease is well defined, both clinically and histologically. It was recognized as a clinical entity over a century ago; effective treatment was installed more or less at the same time. Few diseases can claim such a long history of prevention.

The following review concerns our present knowledge of the disease.

CLINICAL COURSE

The onset usually occurs in the first 12 months of life. However, the very early stages of the disease, when a tumour of less than 1 mm is present, are only observed in familial cases because in such cases extensive ophthalmological investigations (retinoscopy) are performed at regular intervals from birth onwards. For this reason, accurate data about the age of onset in general cannot be given. In figure 1 the age at which the disease was first discovered in 48 patients is plotted against the severity.

Most of the sporadic cases only become manifest after the tumour has grown to a considerable size in at least one eye. The tumour can then be seen as a *white pupillary* reflex, or, when it involves or covers the central retinal area, manifests itself by the development of a *strabismus*. Except in very rare cases of regression, if untreated the disease leads to death by intracranial extension or general metastasis of the tumour.

Because the intracranial extension of the tumour usually occurs late, the enucleation of one or, if indicated, both eyes was the life-saving therapy until approximately 1935. In an attempt to avoid the enucleation of both eyes, radiotherapy or thermal destruction of the tumour (originally by diathermy,

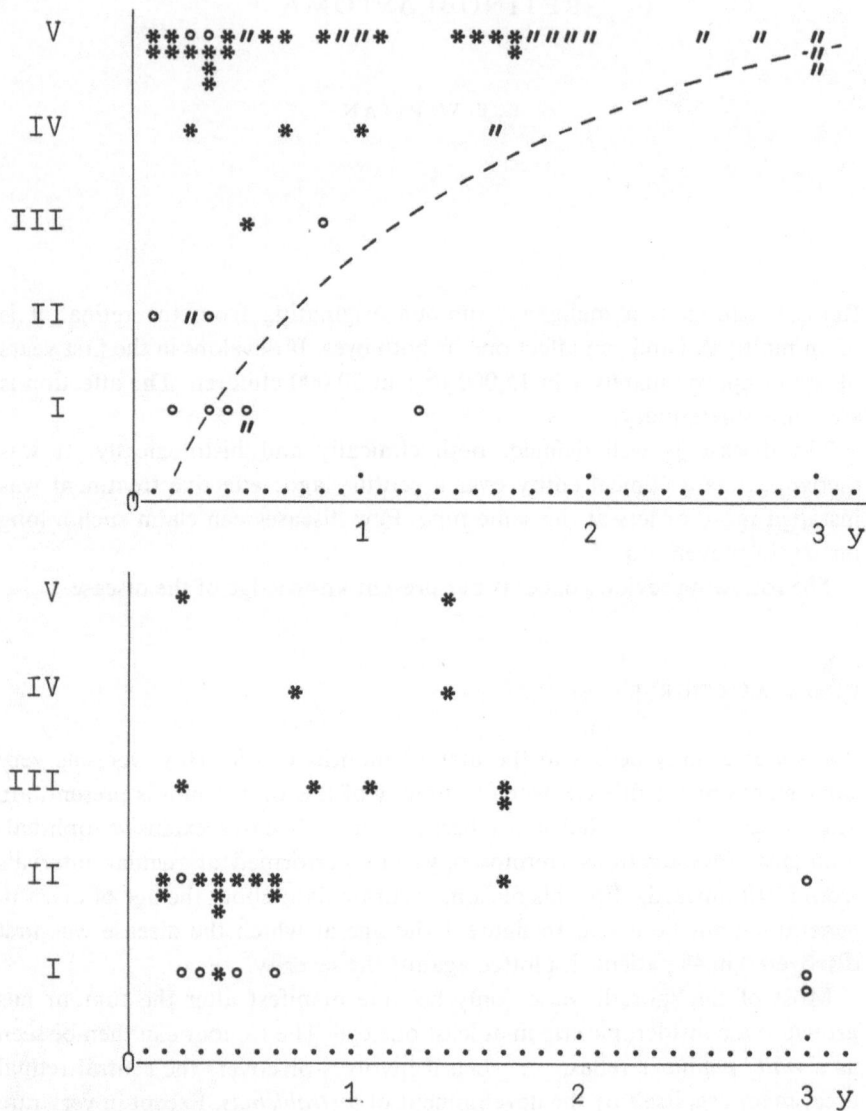

Fig. 1. *Age at which retinoblastoma is detected plotted against the Reese classification of severity.*
Top: The 'worst' eye
Bottom: The 'best' eye
″   Unilateral sporadic
*   Bilateral sporadic
°   Hereditary

later by light- and cryo-coagulation) has been performed. In this way at least some visual acuity has occasionally been preserved. Although this so-called 'conservative treatment' undoubtedly carries a certain risk, the benefits are generally considered to outweigh the risks.

PATHOLOGIC ANATOMY

Microscopically the tumour consists of undifferentiated cells showing regionally a primitive organization in the form of globular structures known as the Wintersteiner rosettes. In these structures the tumour seems to form small retinal cups which supports its supposed origin from the primordial cells of the retina, the retinoblasts. Extensive areas of necrosis may occur and calcium compounds are often deposited in these areas.

A number of growth types can be distinguished. When the tumour arises in the inner layers of the retina it will grow into the vitreous cavity. This is called the *endophytic* growth type.

When the tumour originates in the outer layers of the retina it will detach the retina from the choroid. This is the *exophytic* growth type. In this second group the prognosis is poorer than in the endophytic type, because the close contact of the tumour with the choroid permits dissemination via the bloodstream and infiltration of the sclera.

In rare cases the tumour shows a diffuse growth pattern infiltrating all layers of the retina. This type has an extremely bad prognosis.

In general, extension of the tumour outside the eye is a relatively late phenomenon.

PRINCIPLES OF PREVENTION

Genetic counseling is the most important factor in the prevention of retino-blastoma. This is evident for the familial cases but also holds for the bilateral sporadic cases. It should, however, also include the unilateral sporadic cases. Although only approximately one-fifth of these individuals will eventually transmit the disease there is as yet no way either on clinical grounds or by laboratory tests to distinguish this group from the 'non-transmitters'. Although it will take at least one generation to produce definite proof, every unilateral sporadic retinoblastoma patient should be considered as a possible genetic case with an average chance of approximately 10% for his or her children to become affected. Due to the high degree of penetrance – between 80 and 100%, possibly varying from family to family – transmission through apparently healthy individuals is unusual. The most likely to be affected are the brothers and sisters of a sporadic retinoblastoma patient. The risk is estimated to be no more than 1 to 4%. In cases of recurrence in a sib one of the parents has in all probability been the carrier of a non-penetrant retinoblastoma gene.

For genetic counseling to be of any use we must be able to recognize sporadic cases of retinoblastoma at a very early stage. This is of extreme importance for minimizing the damage in the affected children, because generally the tumour grows rapidly and the chances of preserving some visual acuity will diminish quickly.

So far, however, the task of early detection seems to be unsolvable. The disease is very rare and few practitioners will have dealt with the problem before. The only way available to us at present to detect a beginning retinoblastoma is by a thorough ophthalmoscopical examination under general anaesthesia. It is obviously impossible – and unjustifiable in view of the risks a general anaesthesia involves at this age – to make this a routine investigation in newborn children. Thus, sporadic cases of retinoblastoma are not generally diagnosed until the first clear symptoms are present. The most frequent symptoms are:

1. A *white pupillary reflex* when the tumour becomes visible behind the pupillary aperture (in 60% of the cases).
2. A *strabismus* when the central retinal area is involved or is covered by the tumour (30%).
3. A diversity of symptoms such as a painful red eye, bleeding or an accumulation of tumour cells in the anterior chamber or pupillary anomalies.

At this advanced stage of the disease a unilateral tumour is almost always beyond the reach of therapy. Fortunately the other eye, if affected at all, is usually in a less advanced stage and might be saved by conservative treatment.

PREVENTION IN THE NETHERLANDS

Genetic counseling has proved to be a very suitable method for the partial prevention of retinoblastoma due to the work of the Netherlands Society for the Prevention of Blindness. For many years this Society has registered nearly all cases of retinoblastoma occurring in The Netherlands, and the archives contain patients from over a hundred years. These individuals are followed throughout their reproductive life and are given advice in connection with marriage and childbirth. However, even the most effective genetic counseling cannot prevent more than a fraction of the total number of retinoblastoma cases and more attention should be paid to the early recognition of sporadic cases.

Although the general medical care in The Netherlands seems to be well developed, cases of retinoblastoma that are not properly diagnosed, in spite of timely recognition of the symptoms by the parents, are still encountered. The rarity of the disease may explain this but should never be considered an adequate excuse, especially in view of the severity of the ensuing symptoms.

I therefore strongly recommend the early referral to an ophthalmologist of children showing one of the two major early symptoms of retinoblastoma, i.e., the white pupillary reflex or strabismus.

AN APPROACH TO THE PROBLEM OF HEREDITARY AND NON-HEREDITARY RETINOBLASTOMA

G. J. P. A. ANDERS

Between 1930 and 1960, 326 infants who developed retinoblastoma were born in The Netherlands. The material discussed here was obtained mainly by analysis and supplementation of the data published by Schappert-Kimmyser *et al.* (1) in 1961. Of the 326 cases, 31 were familial and 295 isolated (sporadic). Familial cases (in our material 25 were bilateral and 6 unilateral) are inherited according to an autosomal dominant pattern of inheritance. Every child of a patient with hereditary bilateral retinoblastoma has a 50 per cent chance of developing the tumour. In cases of familial unilateral retinoblastoma the predisposition is transmitted in the same way but the morbidity risk is distinctly lower, i.e., about 70 per cent of that of the former group (2).

The sporadic cases in the above-mentioned series fall into two groups: bilateral tumours (29 per cent) and unilateral tumours (71 per cent). The bilateral sporadic cases can be considered to arise from new mutations. They will therefore be inheritable. For the unilateral sporadic cases it is known from extensive research that only a limited proportion concern a hereditary form, the estimates varying from 1 to 20 per cent (2). The others arise by somatic changes. Even if one chooses for the highest percentage, 57% of sporadic retinoblastomas in our material will be non hereditary.

Many attempts have been made to explain the occurrence of both hereditary and non-hereditary forms of retinoblastoma. Two highly divergent theories have been formulated. One of these concerns the mutational origin of all kinds of retinoblastoma. Knudson (3) published a very extensive analysis of this kind. According to him, all hereditary retinoblastomas are based on a gametic mutation followed by an isolated mutation in a single cell, and the non-hereditary cases arise from two parallel somatic mutations in the same retinal cell (2). The other theory was put forward by Vogel, who argues that the non-hereditary forms are phenocopies of the dominant autosomal hereditary type (4).

A contribution to the solution of the problem of the nature of the anomaly promoting the development of retinoblastoma has, however, been provided rather unexpectedly from the part of cytogenetics.

Since 1963, more than 40 patients have been described who showed various physical abnormalities such as aplasia or hypoplasia of the thumb and microcephalia and in whom a deletion was observed in a group D chromosome. Approximately one-fourth of these patients also had retinoblastoma. These patients are now known to have a defect of band 3 in 13q (5). On the basis of this finding it seems possible that the gene mutation underlying the hereditary form of retinoblastoma is a deficiency mutation. If the gene in question regulates the synthesis not of an enzyme but of a structural protein for instance, a deficiency of this kind could be expressed as a gene dosage effect. It would then be mainly a matter of cell differentiation and threshold values whether, and if so where, the deficiency resulting from the mutation would lead to a manifest anomaly. Compared with Knudson's mutation theory, this hypothesis has the advantage that for the realization of a genetically caused retinoblastoma fewer mutation steps are necessary. The genesis of phenocopies of the hereditary form of retinoblastoma also becomes understandable in the light of this interpretation. When an abnormality is caused by the lack of a particular substance, this deficiency can in principle arise from either endogenous (genetic) or exogenous (milieu) factors. Furthermore, the fact that, as recently demonstrated by Kitchin and Elsworth (6), patients with a proven hereditary bilateral retinoblastoma have a distinctly greater chance of developing additional tumours than patients with the unilateral sporadic form, is more easily explained by this hypothesis than by the mutation theory.

The occurrence of gene mutations is most probably determined by factors of a very complex nature whose only specific feature is that they induce changes in the DNA. In view of this highly complex causality, important and abrupt fluctuations in the frequency of spontaneous mutations are in general not to be expected, particularly with respect to individual genes. Phenocopies, on the other hand, arise from specific disturbances occurring between the formation of the primary product of a given gene and the ultimate formation of the corresponding trait. Such conditions are not liable to be met frequently but if some exogenous agent turns out to be capable of disturbing a particular phenotypic pathway, the frequency of the corresponding phenocopy is apt to rise considerably. It may therefore be expected that the frequency of phenocopies of a given mutation will be subject to much greater fluctuations than that of the mutation itself. Thus if retinoblastoma can be the result of both mutation and phenocopy, major frequency fluctuations would, other conditions of genetic equilibrium remaining unchanged, occur from the formation of phenocopies rather than by mutagenesis. We made an attempt to find out whether this was the case in the Dutch retinoblastoma material.

If the annual frequency figures of sporadic retinoblastoma in The Netherlands between 1931 and 1960 are compared, an appreciable variability is found. But if a distinction is made between bilateral and unilateral tumours, the bilateral show much less variability and a normal distribution ($p > 0.50$, Shapiro and Wilk's test), whereas the unilateral tumours, tested in the same way, are not normally distributed ($p < 0.01$) (7). The ratio between the lowest and highest frequency per year is $1:6.8$ for the bilateral cases and $1:8.6$ for the unilateral cases. (The year 1942, in which no bilateral cases were found, was not included in the calculation of these ratios.) The unilateral tumours show a striking concentration of high frequencies between 1945 and 1955, a concentration which was not observed in the case of the bilateral material. Application of van Eeden's test (8) showed a significant ($p < 0.05$) tendency for the annual frequencies of unilateral sporadic tumours to increase between 1934 and 1960; this was not demonstrable to the same degree for the bilateral tumours. Trend tests are difficult to interpret, and we therefore wish to reserve comment until a more thorough statistical analysis of the entire material has been completed. Nevertheless such data could make it worth-while to do further research on the basis of the hypothesis that retinoblastoma is not only the result of a mutagenic process but that a large number of these tumours arise as phenocopies. If exogenous factors should prove to play an important part in the occurrence of a large number of retinoblastomas, our approach to prevention, and prevention itself, would need a form very different from that which we had to choose if the tumours were interpreted on a purely genetic basis.

ACKNOWLEDGEMENTS

The material discussed above is mainly due to the incessant and devoted efforts of Dr. Schappert-Kimmyser helped by Drs. R. Nijland under the auspices of the Dutch General Association for Prevention of Blindness. Drs. R. P. Wegener helped with sorting out and checking many data. Drs. H. J. Bronts, Prof. Dr. W. Schaafsma and Dr. G. N. van Vark gave very useful suggestions for the statistical evaluation of the material.

REFERENCES

1. Schappert-Kimmyser, J., G. D. Hemmes and R. Nijland, The heredity of retinoblastoma. *Ophthalmologica 151*, 197 (1961).
2. Briard-Guillemot, M. L., C. Bonaïti-Pellié, J. Feingold and J. Frézal, Etude génétique du rétinoblastome. *Humangenetik 24*, 271 (1974).
3. Knudson, A. G., Jr., Mutation and cancer: statistical study of retinoblastoma. *Proc. nat. Acad. Sci. (Wash.) 68*, 820 (1971).
4. Vogel, F., Neue Untersuchungen zur Genetik des Retinoblastomas (Glioma retinae). *Z. menschl. Vererb.-u Konstit.-Lehre 34*, 205 (1957).
5. Wilson, M. G., J. W. Towner and Atsuko Fujimoto, Retinoblastoma and D-chromosome Deletions. *Amer. J. hum. Genet. 25*, 57 (1973).
6. Kitchin, F. D. and R. M. Ellsworth, Pleiotropic effects of the gene for retinoblastoma. *Journal of Medical Genetics 11*, 244 (1974).
7. Shapiro, S. S. and M. B. Wilk, An analysis of variance test for normality (complete samples). *Biometrika 52*, 591 (1965).
8. Rümke, Chr. L. and C. van Eeden, *Statistiek voor medici*. Leiden 1961.

DISCUSSION

PAPER OF G. J. P. A. ANDERS

Mrs. Sachs: Are patients with retinoblastoma routinely screened for chromosomal diagnosis?

Anders: No, and it is not expected to be a useful approach.

SCREENING FOR PHENYLKETONURIA

W. M. J. VAN DUYNE

INTRODUCTION

In 1966, the then State-Secretary of Social Affairs and Public Health appointed a study group to provide advice on the desirability of early detection of phenylketonuria patients and the feasibility of a screening program in The Netherlands. In 1970, this study group submitted its final report (1), in which the conclusion was reached that mass screening for phenylketonuria of infants in the second week after birth was desirable and organizationally feasible in The Netherlands. This conclusion was based in part on the results of two investigations into phenylketonuria performed in The Netherlands during this period.

One of these studies consisted of a pilot screening of newborns in the provinces of Groningen and Friesland, the other of a survey of phenylketonuria patients in institutions for the mentally retarded. A number of aspects of these studies will be discussed in this report, with special attention to the elements which influenced the decision to apply the screening of newborns for phenylketonuria as a routine procedure on a national scale before the end of 1974.

Phenylketonuria belongs to the group of recessively inherited metabolic diseases. The clinical picture was first described by Fölling in 1934, and has since been the subject of many publications. The disease is characterized by the absence of L-phenylalanine-hydroxylase in the liver, as a result of which the amino acid phenylalanine is not converted into tyrosine or only in very small amounts. This gives rise to anomalous degradation products of phenylalanine, which are assumed to lead to mental deficiency. When this metabolic defect is detected in time – preferably as soon as possible after the first week of life – the institution of a phenylalanine-poor diet can prevent mental retardation, and normal development of the infant is possible.

In addition to the classical phenylketonuria other – atypical and transient – forms of hyperphenylalaninaemia have been distinguished, which complicated the diagnostic and therapeutic criteria. For a more detailed description of phenylketonuria, reference is made to the extensive literature (for a short review in Dutch, see the recent G.H.I. bulletin) (2).

Interest in phenylketonuria became broader in the 1960s with the development of new laboratory techniques by which an elevation of the phenylalanine level in the blood could be demonstrated easily and reliably. The best known of these is the Guthrie test (3), a microbiological method suitable for large-scale application. Screening programs were then carried out in various countries and large numbers of newborns were investigated for phenylketonuria. In this context it will be useful to examine the concept screening.

THE GENERAL BASIS OF SCREENING

The purpose of screening is the detection of individuals who *probably* suffer from a given disease in a stage in which treatment or correction can still be effective (4). Thus, screening is a form of secondary prevention which is concerned with the pre-symptomatic phase of a disease (or unrecognized symptomatic disease) and is in principle limited to the selection of individuals who should undergo further investigation for definitive diagnosis.

The decision to adopt screening for a given disease as a country-wide provision must be weighed carefully. The most important general principles on which the decision can be based, may be formulated as follows:

1. The disease to be detected must be sufficiently important in relation to public health as a whole. Here, the concepts severity and frequency of the affection predominate.
2. The natural course of the disease must be adequately known, and the disease must be curable or the course reversible. With respect to phenylketonuria – and certainly the classical form – this condition can be said to be satisfied, although certain aspects of the dietary treatment are still uncertain, for instance the duration of application of the diet.
3. Adequate facilities must be available for the definite diagnosis of the individuals indicated by the screening as potential patients, and this also holds for any treatment that might be required. Since phenylketonuria is a very rare disease, this condition is not a problem in the situation prevailing in The Netherlands.
4. The method chosen for the screening must satisfy high standards of speci-

ficity and sensitivity. These concepts can be illustrated by the following scheme:

test result	actual condition	
	affected	non affected
—	c	d
+	a	b

specificity $= \dfrac{d}{d + b}$,   this fraction thus being determined by the relationship between d and b, which makes it a measure for the percentage of false-positive results.

sensitivity $= \dfrac{a}{a + c}$,   which gives the percentage of false-negative results.

Both the specificity and the sensitivity are highly dependent on the distribution of a variable of measurement over the population. In principle, two types of distribution can be expected, one characterized by a single peak and the other by two peaks (fig. 1a and 1b).

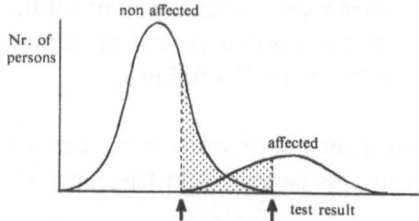 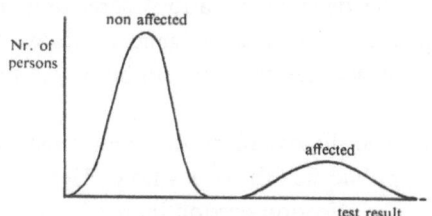

Fig. 1a. Bimodal distribution with area of overlap.   *Fig.* 1b. Bimodal non-overlapping distribution.

False-negative and false-positive results will be found in the overlapping or transitional areas; the choice of the upper limit for a possible positive result will have an influence on the ratio false-negative to false-positive. A disjunct two-peak distribution (fig. 1b) of a variable with minimal false-positive and false-negative results is thus favourable for screening. The phenylalanine content of the blood in classical phenylketonuria approaches this situation after the first week of life.

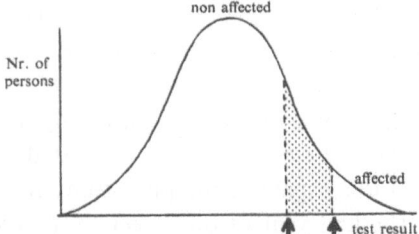

Fig. 2. Unimodal distribution with a transitional area.

5. The investigation must be acceptable for the population. Participation in a screening will in principle be voluntary; to achieve adequate motivation for participation in the investigation, the provision of good information is imperative. It is conceivable that an investigation felt to be unpleasant could influence the degree of participation; in the present case the heel-prick for collecting a blood sample from the infant might lead to emotional objections on the parents' part. Important information on this point was provided by the pilot study performed in Groningen and Friesland, which will be discussed below.

6. The administrative and organizational element of mass screening must be adequately planned, and should burden the groups involved in its execution as little as possible.

7. The cost of the screening must be quantifiable as well as acceptable in terms of the savings that can be expected from the effect aimed at (cost-benefit analysis).

THE PILOT SCREENING IN GRONINGEN AND FRIESLAND

This pilot study was initiated by the study group on phenylketonuria and was instituted after consultation between the governmental body for the state supervision of public health and several provincial health-care organizations. The organization and execution of the screening was placed in the hands of the provincial Maternal and Child Health Care Services. The preparations were made in 1967, and the program was fully applied in both provinces in 1968. The main purpose of this pilot study was to obtain an impression of the organizational feasibility of a screening program intended to test the blood of all liveborn children in these provinces, preferably in the second week after birth.

The method chosen for the investigation, as mentioned above, was the

Guthrie test, a microbiological semi-quantitative determination of the phenylalanine content of the blood. This laboratory test was done in the regional laboratories selected for participation.

Detailed records of the course of the screening program were maintained according to a predetermined scheme, which permitted evaluation. Several detailed publications on this aspect of the pilot study have appeared (1, 5). Because the results of the first year of the screening (1968) were taken as a basis for the report of the study group on phenylketonuria (1), some relevant data from that year are included here. The continuation of the screening in 1969 and the following years did not show any essentially new aspects.

The answer to the most important question, i.e., whether a sufficiently large number of newborns could be included in the study, is indicated by Table 1.

Table 1. Percentage of participation in phenylketonuria screening in 1968.

		Groningen	Friesland
Liveborn children	n =	9,579	10,010
Investigated children		98.2	98.1
Parental refusal		0.8	0.6
Other reasons for non-participation		1.0	1.3

In both provinces the percentage of participation was over 98, and refusal accounted for less than 1 per cent of all newborns. This shows very clearly that the organization of the screening was highly effective and also that it was accepted by virtually the entire population. The results are even more impressive in view of the fact that in these provinces in 1968 the majority of the deliveries occurred at home.

Table 2. Blood sampling, phenylketonuria screening 1968.

		%
Home delivery	district nurse	85.8
(n = 12, 182)	family physician	9.0
	midwife	4.2
	maternity-centre	1.0
		100.0
Hospital delivery	nurse	78.2
(n = 7,016)	lab. technician	19.3
	physician	1.5
	other	1.1
		100.0

With respect to the organization of the screening it is of particular interest to know for the home deliveries who performed the heel-prick for the collection of the blood sample. At the beginning of the project it was agreed that if so desired the family physician could leave the sampling to the district nurse or the midwife.

It is evident from Table 2 that for the home deliveries the blood sampling was done mainly by the district nurse (86%). This tendency on the part of the family doctors to leave the sampling to the district nurse was found to increase in the following years.

One of the important questions related to the study was whether the blood sampling could be performed as soon as possible after the first week. Analysis of a 10 per cent sample performed in Friesland in 1968 gave the results shown in Table 3.

Table 3. Time of blood sampling 1968, Friesland (n = 1,000).

Days after birth	%
7-14	94.4
15-21	3.8
22-28	0.9
29-42	0.7
43>	0.2
	100.0

A similar sample analysed for Groningen in 1969 showed that 98 per cent of the blood samples were collected in the second week after birth, so that it may be concluded that the ideal age for the test was very closely approached.

The results of the Guthrie test are shown in Table 4.

Table 4. Results of pilot screening for phenylketonuria 1968.

		%
Guthrie test	negative	99.40
(n = 19,198)	dubious	0.07
	positive	0.01
	too little material	0.50
	Total	100.00

Values above 4 mg phenylalanine per 100 ml were considered positive and those between 2 and 4 mg dubious. Repetition of the test on the basis of dubious or (false)-positive results which was required in 16 cases out of the 19, 198 proved to be negative in all. This ratio seems completely acceptable. The repetition of a test for phenylketonuria, which implies the possibility of the existence of a very serious disease, can easily cause panic in the parents, which means that in these cases good communication between them and the physician in question is imperative. Especially because the further investigation of children with a positive or dubious result in the Guthrie test usually occurs in hospital, it is highly relevant that this number forms only a small fraction of the total number of infants investigated.

PHENYLKETONURIA PATIENTS AMONG INSTITUTIONALIZED MENTAL DEFECTIVES

A survey of all phenylketonuria patients in institutions for the mentally retarded on 1 January 1968 was also initiated by the study group. For this survey the Chief Inspector of Mental Health requested the cooperation of the boards of directors and heads of all institutions and residential homes in The Netherlands for a screening of all their current inmates by means of the Guthrie test. At the conclusion of the survey, 22,493 mental defectives had been investigated, which closely approximates the estimate of 23,000 institutionalized cases at that time.

During the investigation, 148 phenylketonuria patients were detected. To obtain more information about these patients, a follow-up questionnaire survey was made with the cooperation of all of the institutions involved (1, 6). The results showed that the 148 patients belonged to 129 families, and that 14 of these families had 2 or more children in institutions (see Table 5).

Table 5. Number of phenylketonuria patients per family.

Nr. of patients per family	Nr. of families	Nr. of patients
1	115	115
2	10	20
3	3	9
4	1	4
Total	129	148

The age of the patients with phenylketonuria living in the institutions on 1-1-1968 varied between 5 and 70 years. It is remarkable that females seem to predominate in the older age groups (Table 6).

A question was included concerning the origin of the 148 patients. Of these, 146 had been born in The Netherlands and the place of birth was known. This made it possible to see whether this material would supply an indication concerning regional differences in the occurrence of phenylketonuria. The results, based on the number of families with phenylketonuria children per province, are shown in Table 7.

Table 6. Mental defectives with phenylketonuria divided according to age and sex.

age	m	f	total
0-4	1	–	1
5-9	9	4	13
10-14	9	18	27
15-19	14	14	28
20-24	15	12	27
25-29	5	3	8
30-34	5	10	15
35-39	3	4	7
40-44	4	3	7
45-49	–	2	2
50-54	2	2	4
55-59	–	3	3
60-64	–	3	3
65>	–	3	3
Total	67	81	148

Table 7. Families with phenylketonuria children, according to the province of birth.

Province	number observed PKU families	number of PKU families expected*	95% confidence intervall**
Groningen	5	5.6	2.2-13.1
Friesland	1	5.4	1.6-11.7
Drenthe	3	3.5	1.1-10.2
Overijssel	9	8.4	4.1-17.1
Gelderland	13	13.6	7.7-23.5
Utrecht	2.5	7.4	2.8-14.4
Noord-Holland	26.5	24.0	15.4-35.7
Zuid-Holland	18	31.4	21.1-44.0
Zeeland	1	3.4	0.6- 8.8
Noord-Brabant	38	14.7	8.4-24.7
Limburg	10	9.0	4.1-17.1
Total	127	127	

* On the basis of the Central Bureau of Statistics census of 1960.
** According to the Poisson distribution.

The results of these calculations must be interpreted cautiously, because they do not include the deceased and the living, non-institutionalized patients. However, the number of families detected in the province of Noord-Brabant is so much higher than the expected number that a higher gene frequency for phenylketonuria in this area is a definite possibility.

The age of the phenylketonuria patients at the (first) admission to an institution was also known, and therefore the mean duration of residence could be calculated for the patients present on 1 January 1968. This amounted to 12.6 years, with a range of 1 to 70 years (see Table 8).

Table 8. Duration of residence and age at admission to an institution (in years).

Age group	Nr. of PKU patients	Mean duration	Mean age at admission
0-9	11	1.9	5.4
10-19	51	7.3	7.3
20-29	34	13.4	9.7
30-39	22	17.2	16.2
40-49	9	15.9	28.1
50-59	7	29.3	24.6
60 and over	6	32.6	32.7
Total	140	12.6	12.5
(unknown)	(8)		

It is striking that those in the higher age groups had been admitted at appreciably older ages than those in the younger age groups. A well-founded explanation for this phenomenon cannot be given on the basis of the available information. It seems, however, that the possibilities for admission may have been more limited formerly than at present. Another assumption, one for which the data offer some support, is that the older patients reach a slightly higher developmental level, which is accompanied by an increased life expectancy.

An attempt was also made in this study to obtain an impression of the severity of the mental retardation in the detected phenylketonuria patients. Since a standardized measurement of the intelligence quotient was not feasible in this situation, preference was given to four questions related to functioning which would at least give some impression of the developmental level, i.e., motor function, performance capacity, speech, and contactual functioning. Each of these functions was scored from 1 to 3, so that the total score of a patient could vary from 4 (very poor) to 12 (reasonably good).

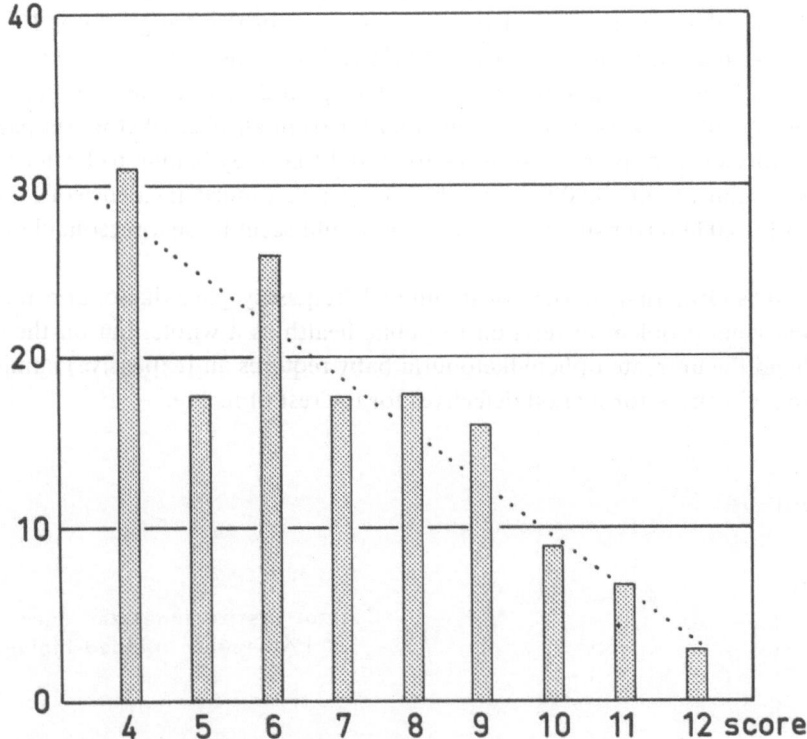

Fig. 3. Developmental level of phenylketonuria patients.

As can be seen from figure 3, the regression line of the total score per patient shows a distinct increase in the number of patients as the score decreases, which indicates that most of these patients belong to the group with a severe degree of mental defectiveness.

DISCUSSION

The two investigations described above supplied arguments in favour of the institution of a nation-wide screening for phenylketonuria. The survey not only yielded the prevalence of institutionalized mental defectives with phenylketonuria (148 on 1 January 1968) but also made it possible to estimate the incidence of phenylketonuria among newborns. It is evident from Table 6 that most of the patients occur in the age group of 10 to 25 years, amounting to 5 to 6 per year class. According to Lang (7), half of the phenylketonuria patients die before the age of 20 and three-quarters before the age of 30 years. If we assume that far from all phenylketonuria patients of this age group are institutionalized and that they belong to birth cohorts averaging about 230,000 in number, a phenylketonuria incidence of 1:10,000 to 1:15,000 births in The Netherlands would seem to be a reasonable estimate.

It is clear that in view of its limited frequency phenylketonuria forms a marginal problem in relation to public health as a whole, but on the other hand the untreated phenylketonuria baby requires an (expensive) admission to an institute for mental defectives for the rest of its life.

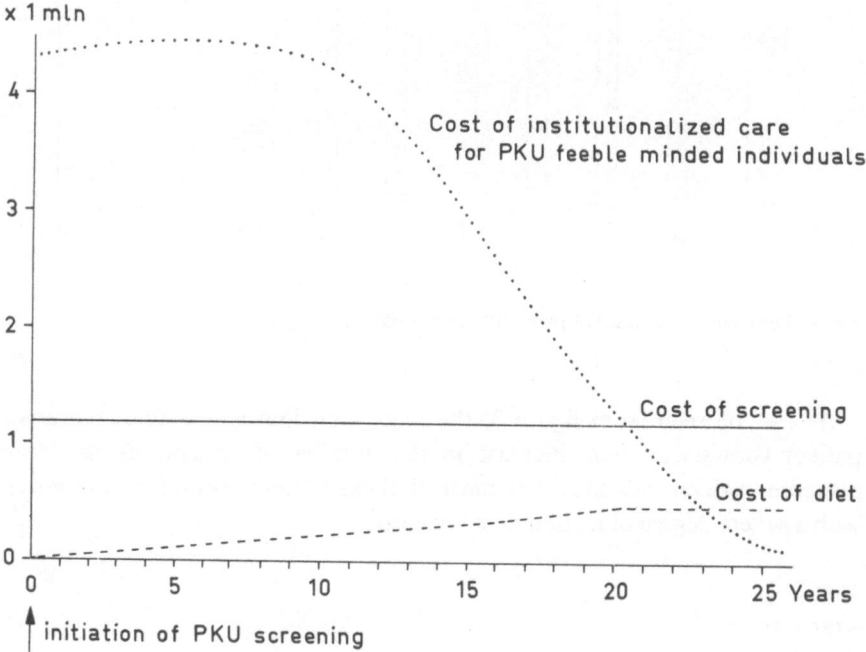

Fig. 4. Time course of the costs in millions of guilders of a nation-wide screening for phenylketonuria, projected over 25 years, in relation to the cost of institutionalization of PKU patients. Dotted line: institution costs; solid line: screening costs; dashed line: diet costs.

The pilot screening in Groningen and Friesland shows unequivocally that screening for phenylketonuria in the situation prevailing in The Netherlands is perfectly feasible, both administratively and organizationally, and in addition is acceptable for the population. The findings in both studies also provide information concerning the financial aspects of this type of screening (see fig. 4).

The curves in figure 4, showing the cost of institutionalization of mental defectives with phenylketonuria, of screening, and of special diets for early detected babies with phenylketonuria are based on price levels prevailing in 1974. The average cost of admission is taken at 80 guilders per day, screening at 6 guilders per test, and extra diet costs ranging from 850 guilders a year for newborns to 1,900 guilders for 5 year olds and older. The maximum duration of the dietary treatment, on which concensus has not been reached, is taken, conservatively, at 20 years. It is evident that some 10 years after the introduction of phenylketonuria screening there will be a rather sharp drop in the expenditure for institutionalization that will more than compensate for the total cost of screening and special diet.

When these findings are evaluated they provide important support for the application of screening. This type of pilot study is indispensable in a period in which the funds available for health care are limited.

REFERENCES

1. *Rapport van de studiegroep fenylketonurie.* Ministerie van Sociale Zaken en Volksgezondheid, 1970.
2. *Phenylketonurie, G.H.I.-bulletin.* Staatstoezicht op de Volksgezondheid, 1974.
3. Guthrie, R. and A. Susi, A simple phenylketonuria screening method for newborn infants. *Pediatrics 32*, 338 (1963).
4. Wilson, J. M. G. and G. Jungner, Principles and practice of screening for disease. *Public Health Paper 34*, W.H.O., 1968.
5. Haverkamp Begemann, N., Screening op phenylketonurie. *T. Soc. Geneesk. 49*, 310 (1971).
6. Anders, G. J. P. *et al.*, The prevalence of phenylketonuria patients in Dutch institutes for the mentally retarded in 1968, *Bulletin v.d. coördinatiecommissie bioch. onderzoek v.d. sectie psych. inst. van de Nat. Ziekenhuisraad 3*, 35 (1973).
7. Lang, K., Phenylpyruvic oligophrenia. *Ergebnisse Inn. Med. u. Kinderheilkunde, 6*, 78 (1955).

DISCUSSION

PAPER OF W. M. J. VAN DUYNE

Veltkamp: PKU-deficient girls should be informed of the risks for their own future pregnancies.

van Duyne: Yes, indeed. Furthermore, when these PKU gene carriers start reproducing, they will double the frequency of homozygotes in the population and multiply the number of heterozygotes by 4 in 70 generations, which is equivalent to 2,000 years.

Galjaard: Would it be feasible, once you know that you are a heterozygote carrier, to have your partner tested?

van Duyne: Yes, it would be possible to concentrate on this group. Registration of heterozygotes is, however, not likely to provide the conclusive answer to the problem of detection of PKU children.

THE EARLY DIAGNOSIS AND PREVENTION OF CYSTIC FIBROSIS

L. P. TEN KATE

INTRODUCTION

Between 1961 and 1965 in the Netherlands 1,239,566 children were born alive (1). Since the frequency at birth of cystic fibrosis was unknown so far in this country, we attempted to reach an estimate on the basis of the number of patients with this disorder in these birth cohorts. To obtain the necessary information, a questionnaire was sent to all pediatricians, lungspecialists and pathologists in The Netherlands. Supplementary data were collected from the Netherlands Foundation for Medical Registration (which registers hospital-admissions), and from the Netherlands Central Bureau of Statistics (which records causes of death). Incidental data were provided by other sources. In this way a total of 342 cases were noticed, which would amount to a frequency of 1 in 3,624 live births.

However, we are not certain about the accuracy of this estimate. On the basis of the information received, the 342 patients could be classified as definite (72 per cent), probable (11 per cent) and possible (17 per cent) cases (fig. 1). The last two of these categories could indicate that not all of the 342 patients really had cystic fibrosis, but they also suggest that, due to inadequate diagnosis, cases might have been missed. Furthermore, it is not certain that the survey traced every patient diagnosed. Of the 342 patients barely 2 per cent were reported by both the participating physicians and the two registries, 37 per cent by two of these three sources and more than 61 per cent by only one of them (fig. 2). The number of unreported patients can only be guessed at. However, completed questionnaires were received from 91.7 per cent of the physicians. Figure 3 shows the geographic distribution of the residences of the 342 patients. Opposite to a relative surplus of patients in the South-Westerly province of the country a relative deficiency of patients may be noticed in the North-Eastern part. The question arises whether these statistically significant differences reflect the actual situation,

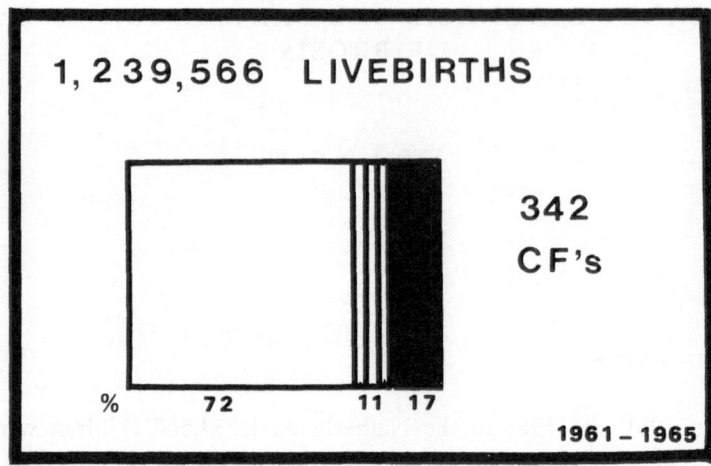

Fig. 1. Results of a retrospective study on the frequency of cystic fibrosis in The Netherlands. For the 342 patients, the white area represents definite cases (72%), the striped area
probable cases (11%), and the black area possible cases (17%).

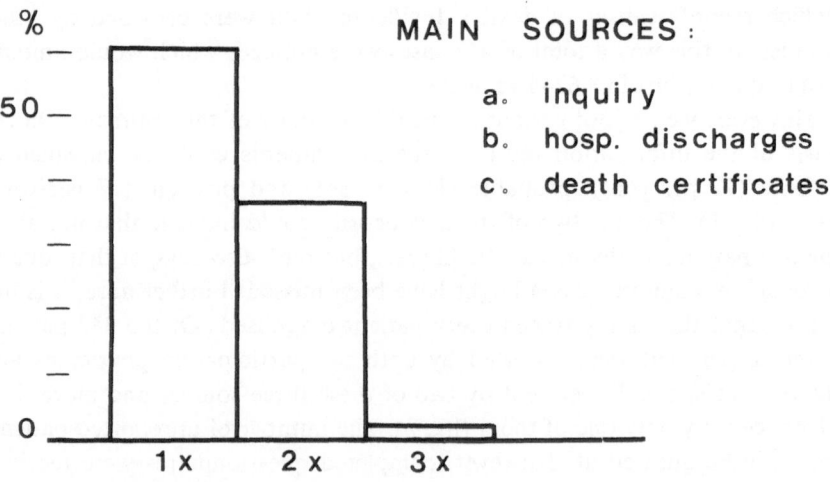

Fig. 2. Multiplicity of ascertainment for 342 cases of cystic fibrosis.

or may be caused by differences in diagnosis or reporting. We have no
special argument in favour of one of these alternatives as yet.

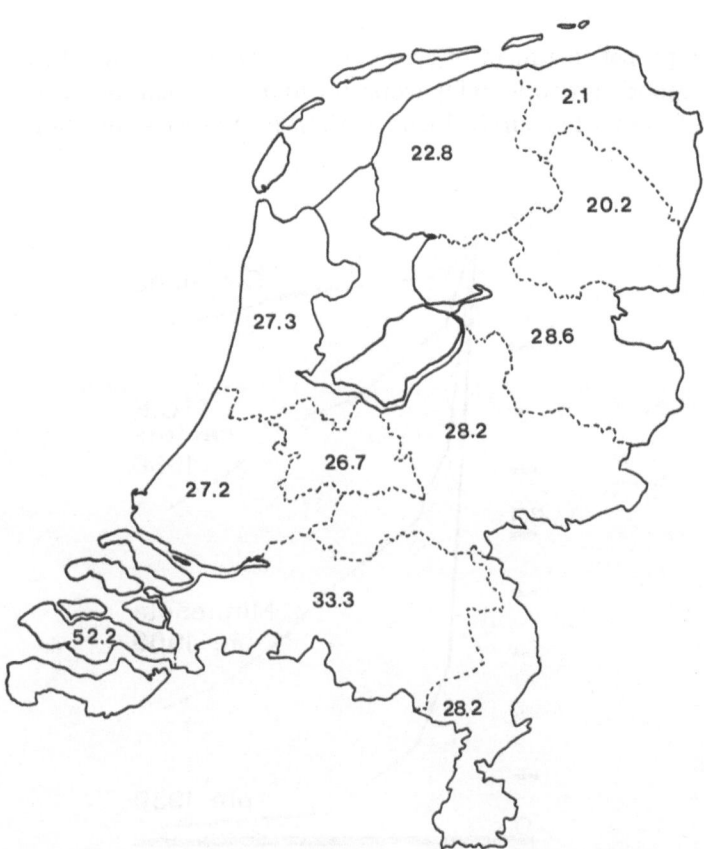

Fig. 3. Geographic distribution of cystic fibrosis in The Netherlands. Number of cases per 100,000 live births (1961-1965).

Certainty about the frequency and geographic distribution of cystic fibrosis in The Netherlands could be obtained by searching the patients more directly, that is by screening methods. Before starting a screening-programme, several questions have to be answered, two of which will be discussed here into some detail. These two questions are: Will screening for cystic fibrosis be of benefit to the patient and/or his family? And secondly, would a screening of this kind be feasible?

THE BENEFIT OF SCREENING FOR CYSTIC FIBROSIS

For the proper treatment of cystic fibrosis, the disease must be recognized. The prognosis is considerably worse for untreated than for treated patients. Figure 4 shows the survival curves given by Warwick and Pogue (2), the

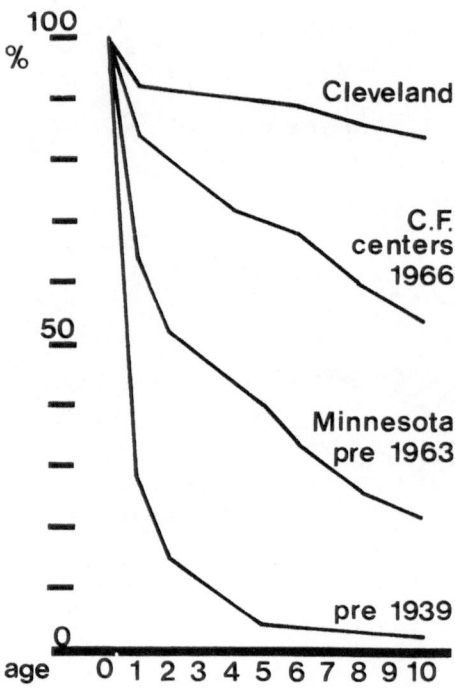

Fig. 4. Cumulative survival curves for cystic fibrosis. Taken from Warwick and Pogue (1968).

data dating from before 1938 corresponding with the situation in which untreated patients find themselves.

The curve pertaining to the prognosis in Minnesota before 1963 reflects conservative treatment of the disease (with antibiotics, pancreatic enzymes, etc.), whereas the curve deriving from hospitals specializing in cystic fibrosis (CF) in 1966 is the result of extension of the treatment to include the pulmonary component (physical therapy, mist tent, etc.). The prognosis in unrecognized cases corresponds best with the pre-1963 situation in Minnesota. Therefore, if screening were to contribute to more frequent recognition of the affection, the prognosis would on average be better for the individual patients.

But screening can also contribute to earlier diagnosis of the disease, even shortly after birth. There are indications that the prognosis of CF is more favourable when the diagnosis is made early. In 1970 Shwachman et al. (3) reported a series of 130 patients in which the diagnosis had been made before the age of three months. These authors found that the patients in whom the diagnosis had been made before the symptoms became manifest had a better prognosis than the children in whom the diagnosis was made during hospitalization. It remains a question, however, whether the latter group must be seen as formed by an unfavourable selection from the main group of patients. In patients diagnosed between 1962 and 1967, Huang et al. (4) found that the prognosis was better when the disease was discovered shortly after birth, before the onset of respiratory symptoms, than in patients first seen between the ages of 2 and 6 months, after the onset of respiratory symptoms. Orenstein et al. (5) compared 25 pairs of CF patients from the same families.

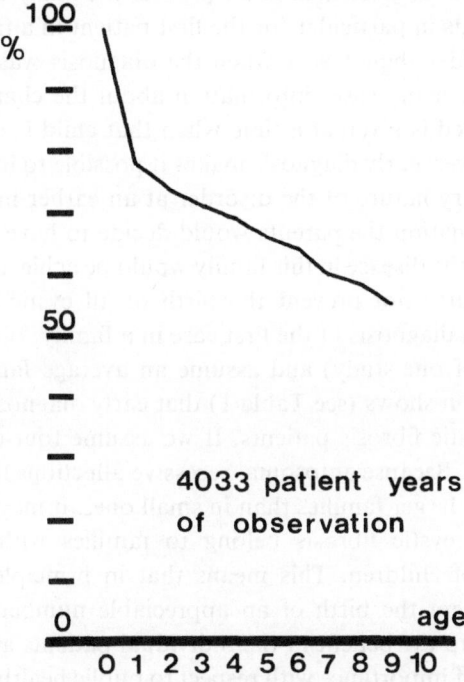

Fig. 5. Longitudinal survival curve for cystic fibrosis patients born between 1961 and 1965 in The Netherlands.

For the youngest patients in the family treatment had been started before the age of one year, but for the older children the average age was $2^8/_{12}$ years. At the age of 7, the younger children showed significantly better scores than their older sibs with respect to a number of parameters for lung function and clinical picture. The survival figures from Cleveland (fig. 4), which according to Warwick and Pogue (2) are based on early prophylactic treatment, also indicate an improvement of the prognosis due to early diagnosis. The survival curve we obtained for the patients born between 1961 and 1965 in The Netherlands (fig. 5) shows a high degree of agreement with the 1966 CF hospital curve and therefore leaves considerable room for improvement.

The early diagnosis of cystic fibrosis benefits the family as well as the patient, because the parents can be informed as soon as possible about the hereditary character of the affection and the consequences for any other children they might have. From figure 6, which shows the distribution of the age at which the diagnosis was made in our series, it is evident that a high proportion of the patients were more than 1 year old when the disease was diagnosed. The data of Orenstein et al. (5) and the analysis of our material show that this holds in particular for the first patient in a family, the majority having been older than 1 year when the diagnosis was made. And this also means that in many cases information about the chance that the next child will be affected is given at a time when that child is on the way or already born. However, early diagnosis makes it possible to inform the parents about the hereditary nature of the disorder at an earlier moment. If on the basis of this information the parents would decide to have no further children, prevention of the disease in this family would be achieved.

This will of course not prevent the birth of all cystic fibrosis patients, since it is based on diagnosis of the first case in a family. If we start with 342 cases (the result of our study) and assume an average family size of three children, calculation shows (see Table 1) that early diagnosis would prevent the birth of 78 cystic fibrosis patients. If we assume four-children families, this number is 108. Because autosomal recessive affections have more chance of being present in larger families than in small ones, it may be assumed that the patients with cystic fibrosis belong to families with more than the average number of children. This means that in principle early diagnosis could indeed prevent the birth of an appreciable number of CF patients. Thus, in addition to the benefit to the individual patients and their families, early diagnosis is of importance with respect to public health.

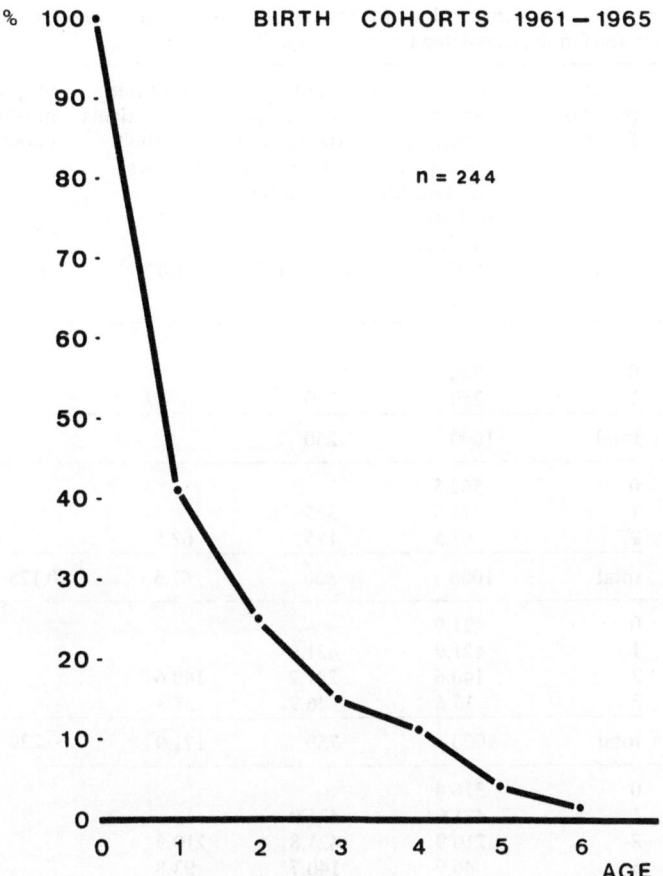

Fig. 6. Estimated percentage of undiagnosed cases of cystic fibrosis in relation to age (on the basis of age at diagnosis in 244 proven cases).

Table 1. Proportion of patients with an autosomal recessive disorder who are not the first such patients in the family, calculated for various family sizes.

nr. of children per family (m)	nr. of patients per family (n)	nr. of families with n patients per 1000 at-risk families with m children (a)*	nr. of patients per 1000 at-risk families with m children (b) = n(a)	nr. of not-first patients per 1000 families (c)**	proportion not-first patients $\dfrac{\varepsilon(c)}{\varepsilon(b)}$
1	0	750			
	1	250	250		
	total	1000	250		
2	0	562.5			
	1	375.0	375		
	2	62.5	125	62.5	
	total	1000	500	62.5	0.125
3	0	421.9			
	1	421.9	421.9		
	2	140.6	281.2	140.6	
	3	15.6	46.9	31.3	
	total	1000	750	171.9	0.229
4	0	316.4			
	1	421.9	421.9		
	2	210.9	421.8	210.9	
	3	46.9	140.7	93.8	
	4	3.9	15.6	11.7	
	total	1000	1000	316.4	0.316

* (a) $= \binom{m}{n} . \frac{1}{4}^n . \frac{3}{4}^{m-n} . 1000$

** (c) $= n(a) - (a)$, with $n \neq 0$

THE FEASIBILITY OF SCREENING FOR CYSTIC FIBROSIS

Bray (6) has reviewed the methods used for screening purposes in cystic fibrosis. We investigated the application of two of these techniques. Since in the Netherlands more than half of the deliveries take place at home (7), we chose the methods based on laboratory analysis of easily obtainable material, which could be sent by post.

We first applied the analysis of nail clippings. In the northern part of the country screening for phenylketonuria has been performed for several years. For this purpose a sample of blood is collected of every newborn in the second week after birth and sent to a central laboratory (8). It seemed likely that the person who took the blood samples could also collect the nail clippings of the same babies.

The nails of patients with cystic fibrosis are characterized by an elevated content of electrolytes, parallelling the increased electrolyte level of the sweat and probably caused by it (9, 10). The electrolyte content of the nails can be determined by chemical or by neutron activation analysis (11, 12). This latter method is to be preferred, because the amount of material available in newborns is very small. Figure 7 shows the results of a study per-

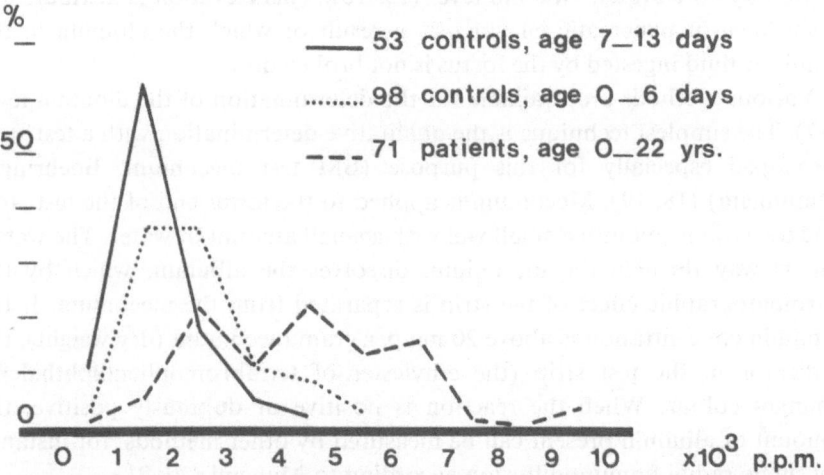

Fig. 7. Sodium concentrations in 151 nail clippings of newborns and 71 nail clippings of cystic fibrosis patients, determined by neutron activation analysis (Netherlands Reactor Centre, Petten).

formed in cooperation with the nuclear reactor centre at Petten (The Netherlands) in 151 nail clippings of newborn babies and 71 from patients with cystic fibrosis.

The material derived from newborns was divided into two groups: samples collected in the first week after birth and samples taken in the second week.

It is clear from figure 7 that: 1) the sodium level in the nails is higher in the first week than in the second; and 2) the values found in the healthy and CF infants overlap to a considerable degree. Both findings are in agreement with

those of other investigators (13). Thus, with this method, at a specificity of
95 per cent we can only expect a sensitivity of 60 per cent. This is disappoint-
ing, particularly in view of the amount of work required for further diagnosis
in the 5 per cent with a positive result. In addition, the rapidity with which
sodium is lost from nails upon contact with water (14) imposes the condition that such contact with water has to be avoided for several hours before
clipping. This forms a great problem for a screening study in which babies
born at home are to be included, since it is impossible to be certain that this
condition has been satisfied.

The second method we explored was the investigation of meconium. It
has long been known that the meconium of healthy newborns has a low
protein content, whereas that of newborns with cystic fibrosis is characterized by an elevated albumin level (15, 16). This elevation is attributed to
a shortage of pancreatic enzymes as a result of which the albumin in the
amniotic fluid ingested by the foetus is not broken down.

Various methods are available for the determination of the albumin level
(17). The simplest technique is the qualitative determination with a test strip
developed especially for this purpose (BM test meconium, Boehringer
Mannheim) (18, 19). Meconium is applied to the lower end of the test strip
and the strip is put into a small vial with a small amount of water. The watei,
on its way through the meconium, dissolves the albumin, which by the
chromatographic effect of the strip is separated from the meconium. If the
albumin concentration is above 20 mg per gram meconium (dry weight), the
indicator in the test strip (the ethylester of tetrabromophenolphthalein)
changes colour. When the reaction is positive or dubiously positive, the
amount of albumin present can be measured by other methods, for instance
by single radial immunodiffusion according to Mancini (20, 21).

The test strip was widely adopted soon after it became available and the
first results obtained in several European countries and the U.S.A. have
been reported. In a random group of 34,300 newborns, 19 cases of cystic
fibrosis, confirmed by sweat test, have been found (22). This amounts to a
frequency of 1 in 1800 live births. Positive results are also obtained when the
albumin level in the meconium is elevated for other reasons (blood, prematurity, intestinal atresia). The total number of positive reactions was less
than 0.5 per cent, which means that the specificity is very high. Although a
few cases of false negative results are already known, the exact sensitivity of
the test is still uncertain.

We have investigated meconium samples from 10,000 newborn infants so
far. These samples werd obtained from hospitals and maternity homes in the

northern part of The Netherlands but also, thanks to the cooperation of the maternity home help of local health-care organizations, from babies born at home. The samples were sent to us by ordinary mail, without refrigeration. The results of the strip test led to the quantitative determination of the albumin content of 233 samples. The criterion applied for this selection was taken very widely and quantification was attempted even when the colour change was minimal. An albumin content of more than 20 mg/g meconium was found in 48 samples (0.48 per cent). The cause of this elevation was found to be prematurity and/or blood contamination in 28 cases and cystic fibrosis in 2 cases (confirmed by pilocarpine iontophoresis). In 18 of the children, no cause for the elevation could be demonstrated (normal by sweat test).

CONCLUSION

On the basis of the foregoing it may be concluded that it is not yet possible to reach a decision for or against the use of meconium screening for the detection of cystic fibrosis. In the first place, more quantitative information about the effect on the prognosis must be obtained. And in the second place, the sensitivity of the method must be reliably determined. Both of these problems will undoubtedly be settled within the next few years, due in part to the international cooperation of such groups as the European working group for cystic fibrosis.

ACKNOWLEDGEMENTS

This investigation was made possible by the support of the Netherlands *Praeventiefonds*, 815 medical specialists, the national medical inspection service, the Central Bureau for Statistics, the Medical Registration Foundation, the Netherlands Cystic Fibrosis Foundation, the Netherlands Reactor Centre, the Paediatric Departments of the University Hospitals in Groningen, Rotterdam and Utrecht, the Obstetrics Department of the Groningen University Hospital, 14 hospitals and maternity homes in the provinces of Groningen, Friesland, Drente and Overijssel and the paediatricians, gynaecologists, general practitioners and midwives attached to them, the maternity home help of Cross organizations in the provinces of Groningen, Friesland and Drente and the firm of Boehringer Mannheim.

REFERENCES

1. C.B.S., *Population and health statistics*, 1965, Maandstatistiek van bevolking en gezondheid 14, 184, 1966.
2. Warwick, W. J. and R. E. Pogue, The prognosis for children with cystic fibrosis based on reasoned approaches to therapy: past, present and future. *J. Asthma Res. 5*, 277-284, 1968.
3. Shwachman, H., A. Redmond and Kon-Taik Khaw, Studies in cystic fibrosis. Report of 130 patients diagnosed under 3 months of age over a 20-year period. *Pediatrics 46*, 335-343, 1970.
4. Huang, N. N., C. N. Macri, J. Girone and A. Sproul, Survival of patients with cystic fibrosis. *Amer. J. Dis. Child. 120*, 289-295, 1970.
5. Orenstein, D. M., T. F. Boat, E. L. Charnock, C. F. Doershuk, R. C. Stern, A. S. Tucker and L. W. Matthews, Early treatment in cystic fibrosis. A sibship study. *Pediat. Res. 7*, 430, 1973.
6. Bray, P. T., *Review of techniques for infant screening*. European Working Group for Cystic Fibrosis, London 1971.
7. C.B.S., *Statistisch Zakboek '73*, 1973.
8. Duyne, W. M. J. van, Phenylketonuria, this book, p. 42.
9. Kopito, L., A. Mahmoodian, R. R. W. Townley, K. T. Khaw and H. Shwachman, Studies in cystic fibrosis. Analysis of nail clippings for sodium and potassium. *New Engl. J. Med. 272*, 504-509, 1965.
10. Grosse, K. P., U. Stephan and F. C. Sitzmann, Untersuchungen über den Natrium- und Kaliumgehalt in Finger- un Zehennägeln. *Z. Kinderheilk. 100*, 87-100, 1967.
11. Babb, A. L., G. L. Woodruff, W. E. Wilson, P. A. Heintz, W. P. Miller and S. J. Stam, The use of neutron activation analysis in the early diagnosis of cystic fibrosis in children. *Trans. Amer. Nuc. Soc. 9*, 591-592, 1966.
12. Kanabrocki, E., L. F. Case, L. A. Graham, T. Fields, Y. T. Oester and E. Kaplan, Neutron-activation studies of trace elements in human fingernail. *J. nucl. Med. 9*, 478-481, 1968.
13. Kollberg, H. and G. Ekbohm, A clinical study of the diagnosis of cystic fibrosis by instrumental neutron activation analysis of sodium in nail clippings. *Acta paediat. Scand. 63*, 411-417, 1974.
14. Kollberg, H. and O. Landström, A methodological study of the diagnosis of cystic fibrosis by instrumental neutron activation analysis of sodium in nail clippings. *Acta paediat. Scand. 63*, 405-410, 1974.
15. Wiser, W. C. and F. R. Beier, Albumin in the meconium of infants with cystic fibrosis: A preliminary report. *Pediatrics 33*, 115-119, 1964.
16. Schachter, H. and G. H. Dixon, A comparative study of the proteins in normal meconium and in meconium from meconium ileus patients. *Canad. J. Biochem. 43*, 381-397, 1965.
17. Prosser, R., H. Owen, F. Bull, B. Parry, J. Smerkinich, H. A. Goodwin and J. Dathan, Screening for cystic fibrosis by examination of meconium. *Arch. Dis. Childh. 49*, 597-601, 1974.
18. Stephan, U., E. W. Busch and R. Dannemann, Ein neuer Screening-Test auf Mukoviszidose. *Pädiat. Prax. 12*, 487-490, 1973.
19. Stephan, U., Testing of meconium of newborns as a screening for cystic fibrosis, In: Mangos, J. A. and R. C. Talamo (ed.), *Fundamental problems in cystic fibrosis and related diseases*. Intercont. Med. Book Corp., New York/London 1973.
20. Bull, F. E., D. E. O. Gladwin and A. D. Griffiths, Immunochemical method for detection of albumin in human meconium. *Arch. Dis. Childh. 49*, 602-605, 1974.
21. Hellsing, K. and H. Kollberg, Analysis of albumin in meconium for early detection of

cystic fibrosis. *Scand. J. clin. Lab. Invest. 33*, 333-340, 1974.
22. Stephan, U., E. W. Busch, H. Kollberg and K. Hellsing, Cystic fibrosis detection by means of test-strip. *Pediatrics 55*, 35-38, 1975.

DISCUSSION

PAPER OF L.P. TEN KATE

Miss van Vooren: Is the frequency difference between various provinces in The Netherlands really significant?

ten Kate: Yes, but we have no ready explanation for this phenomenon.

Muller: Cystic fibrosis is reported to occur frequently without any aberration of the digestive tract but with severe aberrations of the lung. Do these children also have a positive meconium test?

ten Kate: This is a cardinal question. It might mean that children with lung complaints in the absence of digestive-tract aberrations might be missed in certain screening programs. However, this problem is not yet clear.

SPHINGOLIPIDOSES*

C. J. EPSTEIN

The sphingolipidoses comprise a group of lysosomal storage diseases resulting from defects in the catabolism of complex sphingolipids. The majority of
these disorders are manifest in early infancy and result in neurologic deterioration and death in the first few years of life. Some, however, may be more
delayed in appearance and may be compatible with survival into adult
years. Recent reviews of the sphingolipidosis have been published by Volk
et al. (1972), Brady (1973), and Brady et al. (1971).

In this discussion we will be concerned with only some of these disorders,
and these include the conditions covered by the eponyms Gaucher's, Niemann-Pick, Krabbe's, Fabry's, and Tay-Sachs disease. I have chosen these
particular sphingolipidoses either because of our own personal experience
with them or because they raise interesting points with regard to the present
approaches toward the detection and therapy of genetic disorders.

Gaucher's disease results from a deficiency of the enzyme β-glucosidase,
which is responsible for cleaving glucose cerebroside (ceramide glucoside)
into glucose and ceramide. This disease can be subdivided into three genetically distinct entities which can be distinguished clinically and enzymologic-
ally. Adult Gaucher's disease, a condition which is most common in the
Jewish population, expresses primarily as hepatosplenomegaly and bone
marrow infiltration. The most severe, infantile form of the disease is characterized by neurological degeneration, hepatosplenomegaly, bone infiltration,
and early death. There is also a juvenile form of the disease which is slower in
its manifestations than the infantile form but is eventually also characterized
by neurologic involvement. Unlike the adult form, neither the infantile nor
the juvenile forms have a special racial distribution.

Recently, we have also seen a group of patients with what appears to
be still another form of Gaucher's disease (E. L. Schneider and C. J. Epstein,

* Supported in part by grants from the National Foundation – March of Dimes, The
National Institute of General Medical Sciences (GM-19,527), and the Maternal and Child
Health Services (Project No. 445).

unpublished). These patients are young children with massive hepatospleno-megaly and severe pulmonary infiltration, but without any of the neurologic-al manifestations of the infantile or juvenile forms of the disorder. It is still not clear whether this represents a new and distinct form of Gaucher's disease or is a phenotypic variant of one of the other types. Although the activity of β-glucosidase is very diminished in cultured fibroblasts, it has not been possible to distinguish this disorder from the others by biochemical analysis.

Niemann-Pick disease also has several clinical forms. The infantile (type A) form is quite similar to Gaucher's disease and results from a severe deficiency of sphingomyelinase, the enzyme which cleaves sphingomyelin into phos-phoryl-choline and ceramide. Like adult Gaucher's disease, infantile Niemann-Pick disease is most commonly found in the Jewish population. Other forms of Niemann-Pick disease occur later in childhood, with or with-out neurologic involvement (groups B and C), and are associated with less severe degrees of sphingomyelinase deficiency. Another form, referred to as Nova Scotia or group D Niemann-Pick disease is primarily characterized by neurologic manifestations but is not associated with any deficiency of sphingomyelinase.

Partial sphingomyelinase deficiency (approximately 18% of control levels) without neurologic manifestations but with splenomegaly has also been ob-served in cases of the sea-blue histiocyte syndrome (Golde et al. 1975). This is a relatively benign condition in which the main features are the enlarge-ment of the spleen and the presence of macrophages or histiocytes with a characteristic sea-blue appearance on staining.

Krabbe's disease or globoid leukodystrophy results from a deficiency of a β-galactosidase which cleaves galactocerebroside into galactose and ceram-ide. The manifestations of this disorder are primarily in the central nervous system, and there is severe gliosis and almost complete absence of myelin. The white matter of the brain and spinal cord show characteristic 'globoid bodies'.

Tay-Sachs disease is yet another neurodegenerative disorder which makes its appearance in early infancy. After a relatively normal period of 3 to 6 months, the infant develops signs of neurologic deterioration and of blind-ness associated with the development of a cherry red spot in the macula. Tay-Sachs disease results from a deficiency of the enzyme hexosaminidase A, the enzyme which cleaves N-acetylgalactosamine from the terminal end of ganglioside GM_2. Like adult Gaucher's disease and infantile Niemann-Pick disease, Tay-Sachs disease is most prevalent in the Ashkenazi Jewish population. In this group, a heterozygote frequency as high as 1 in 30 to 1 in 35 has been observed, and this corresponds to a homozygote or disease frequency of approximately 1 in 3500 to 1 in 5000. In the non-Jewish population the gene frequency is approximately 10 times less and the resulting disease frequency 100 times less.

Because of the high gene frequency in a small but well defined population, Tay-Sachs disease has proven to be an excellent candidate for population screening for heterozygote detection. Such screening can now be carried out by automated analysis of serum hexosaminidase A and B levels (Delvin et al. 1974). Several screening programs aimed at the Jewish population have already been implemented in the United States and have been directed principally at married couples in the child-bearing ages. If it is found that both the husband and wife are carriers of the gene for hexosaminidase A deficiency, then they are counseled accordingly and are offered the opportunity of an amniocentesis and prenatal diagnosis for Tay-Sachs disease in the event of a subsequent pregnancy (O'Brien 1973). The great acceptance that has been accorded to the Tay-Sachs screening program has been the result of several factors. These include the accuracy, simplicity, and low cost of the test and the availability of amniocentesis so that those at risk can be relieved of the burden of having an affected child.

Fabry's disease results from a deficiency of an α-galactosidase which cleaves the terminal galactose from ceramide trihexoside. Unlike all of the disorders mentioned above which are inherited in an autosomal recessive manner, Fabry's disease is inherited as an X-linked disorder. This leads to much more severe involvement in males than females, although females can develop the disorder. Fabry's disease also differs from the other sphingolipidoses in that it makes its appearance in late childhood or adult life and is characterized by the appearance of reddish-purple keratotic papules over the lower parts of the body and trunk. The scrotum is frequently involved in males. Associated with these skin lesions (angiokeratomas) are severe episodes of burning pain and crises of fever. Kidney disease is a common complication and frequently results in death, in females as well as males.

In recent years there has been considerable interest in possible methods of treating Fabry's disease. Early attempts at the infusion of the missing enzyme produced only transient effects and did not appear to promise long term benefits. However, because of renal failure, several patients with Fabry's disease have received kidney transplants. Somewhat unexpectedly, many of these patients have been documented as having not only improvement in their renal status as a direct result of the new kidney, but also in their subjective complaints – particularly those relating to pain and other crises (Desnick et al. 1972). There is presently considerable dispute about the mechanism by which these beneficial effects are produced, and it has been variously suggested that the benefits result from either the release of enzyme into the circulation, the clearing of the non-metabolized ceramide trihexoside by circulation through the kidney, or by a lessened destruction of red cells which are presumed to be the principal source of the enzyme substrate (Clarke et al. 1972; Krivit et al. 1972). So far, Fabry's disease has been the only one of the sphingolipidoses for which a potentially useful method of treatment has been suggested.

Reference has already been made to the prenatal diagnosis of Tay-Sachs disease. Similar possibilities also exist for many of the other sphingolipidoses, since the enzymes of interest are present within cultured amniotic fluid cells. The genetics group in San Francisco has had direct experience with the prenatal diagnosis of three of the sphingolipidoses, infantile Gaucher's disease, Niemann-Pick disease type A, and Krabbe's disease. In each case, the family presented for prenatal diagnosis after the death of an affected child. Each family was handled in a similar way, in that they first received genetic counseling with regard to the risks of recurrence of the disorder in question as well as of the risks and other complications of the amniocentesis and prenatal diagnosis procedure. Once it was decided that prenatal diagnosis would be undertaken, an amniocentesis was performed at the appropriate time and the amniotic fluid cells cultured by the standard methods (Epstein et al. 1972). Since all of the enzyme assays were carried out by conventional (not micro) assay procedures it was necessary to grow up relatively large quantities of amniotic fluid cells, a process which took as long as 4 or 5 weeks. Control cultures were always grown in parallel with the cultures from the subjects at risk and all samples were submitted and analysed in a blind fashion. In each case, it was possible to document the virtual or complete absence of the enzyme in question, with normal levels of other enzymes assayed as controls (Epstein et al. 1971; Suzuki et al. 1971; Schneider et al. 1972a). On the first attempt, each of the 3 fetuses at risk for the sphingolipid disorders mentioned above was found to be affected and therapeutic abortions were performed. In the case of the parents of the fetuses with Gaucher's and Niemann-Pick disease, another pregnancy was subsequently undertaken and repeat amniocentesis and prenatal diagnosis demonstrated the fetuses to be unaffected.

In each instance in which an abortion was carried out, it was possible to confirm the diagnosis by enzyme studies on tissues from the abortus, biochemical analysis of the fetal organs, and by ultrastructural and conventional histochemical analysis of the fetal tissues (Schneider et al. 1972a, 1972b; Ellis et al. 1973). In all cases it was of interest to observe that there was ultramicroscopic evidence of lipid storage, even in tissues obtained from abortuses less than 20 weeks of gestational age. These findings indicate that the pathological processes resulting from the storage of sphingolipids begin quite early in gestational life and may potentially produce irreversible damage even prior to the time of birth. A similar pathologic picture has also been observed in cases of Tay-Sachs disease and of other sphingolipidoses aborted after prenatal diagnosis.

Despite their relative rarity, except in specific ethnic groups, the sphingolipidoses have played an important role in elucidating the normal metabolism of complex lipids. In addition, they have demonstrated, perhaps more clearly than any other group of biochemical disorders, the great power and resulting benefits of prenatal diagnosis and selective abortion. Lastly, this group of disorders has provided an interesting challenge to those who are interested in developing methods for treatment of genetic disease, although there is a strong (but still unproven) possibility that irreversible damage is done early in the development of fetuses with the infantile neurodegenerative forms of the sphingolipidoses.

REFERENCES

1. Brady, R. O., The abnormal biochemistry of inherited disorders of lipid metabolism. *Fed. Proc. 32:* 1660-1666 (1973).
2. Brady, R. O., W. G. Johnson and B. W. Uhlendorf, Identification of heterozygous carriers of lipid storage diseases. Current status and clinical applications. *Amer. J. Med. 51:* 423-431 (1971).
3. Clarke, J. T. R., R. D. Guttmann, L. S. Wolfe, J. G. Beaudoin and D. D. Morehouse, Enzyme replacement therapy by renal allotransplantation in Fabry's disease. *New Eng. J. Med. 287:* 1215-1281 (1972).
4. Delvin, E., A. Pottier, C. R. Scriver and R. J. M. Gold, The application of an automated hexosaminidase assay to genetic screening. *Clin. Chim. Acta 53:* 135-142 (1974).
5. Desnick, R. J., R. L. Simmons, K. Y. Allen, J. E. Woods, C. F. Anderson, J. S. Najarian and W. Krivit, Correction of enzymatic deficiencies by renal transplantation: Fabry's disease. *Surgery 72:* 203-211 (1972).
6. Ellis, W. G., E. L. Schneider, J. R. McCulloch, K. Suzuki and C. J. Epstein, Fetal globoid cell leukodystrophy (Krabbe's disease). *Arch. Neurol. 29:* 253-257 (1973).
7. Epstein, C. J., R. O. Brady, E. L. Schneider, R. M. Bradley and D. Shapiro, In utero diagnosis of Niemann-Pick disease. *Amer. J. Hum. Genet. 23:* 533-535 (1971).
8. Epstein, C. J., E. L. Schneider, F. A. Conte and S. Friedman, Prenatal detection of genetic disorders. *Amer. J. Hum. Genet. 24:* 214-226 (1972).
9. Golde, D. W., E. L. Schneider, D. F. Bainton, R. O. Brady, C. J. Epstein and M. J.

Cline, Pathogenesis of one variant of sea-blue histiocytosis. Submitted for publication (1975).

10. Krivit, W., R. J. Desnick, R. W. Bernlohr, F. Wold, J. S. Najarian and R. L. Simmons, Enzyme transplantation in Fabry's disease. *New Engl. J. Med. 287:* 1248-1249 (1972).

11. O'Brien, J. S., Tay-Sachs disease: from enzyme to prevention. *Fed. Proc. 32:* 191-199 (1973).

12. Schneider, E. L., W. G. Ellis, R. O. Brady, J. R. McCulloch and C. J. Epstein, Infantile (type II) Gaucher's disease: In utero diagnosis and fetal pathology. *J. Pediat. 81:* 1134-1139 (1972a).

13. Schneider, E. L., W. G. Ellis, R. O. Brady, J. R. McCulloch and C. J. Epstein, Prenatal Niemann-Pick disease: biochemical and histologic examination of a 19-gestational week fetus. *Pediat. Res. 6:* 720-729 (1972b).

14. Suzuki, K., E. L. Schneider and C. J. Epstein, In utero diagnosis of globoid cell leukodystrophy (Krabbe's disease). *Biochem. Biophys. Res. 45:* 1363-1366 (1971).

15. Volk, B. W., M. Adachi and L. Schneck, The pathology of sphingolipidoses. *Semin. Hematol. 9:* 317-348 (1972).

DISCUSSION

PAPER OF C. J. EPSTEIN

Went: Could you offer any suggestions for the remarkable incidence of quite a number of these lipidoses representing related functions in the Ashkenazim Jewish population from different areas in Poland and Russia? It seems hardly possible that it could only be due to chance.

Epstein: Well, the conventional explanation of such a high incidence of any one specific disorder is usually called the founder effect, i.e. that a given individual in a small population has such a mutation and this then spreads through a fairly restricted group, but as the group enlarges the number of individuals carrying the gene increases. That would explain any one of the three. I think your question of why three different ones occur in the same population is an interesting one, and I have no answer for that. I do not know whether any one has an answer. Various disorders affect various specific ethnic groups, but I do not know of any other group which has this type of picture. Whether there are – and perhaps that is implicit in your question – also selective factors that have operated within these populations to maintain the frequency of these genes at some higher level – whether that could be possible – again, I do not know. It would be intriguing to investigate although I do not know what selective factors operate in the Eastern European Jewish population.

Anders: Do you have any false negatives in your tests on heterozygotes or do you have some variabilities in these tests?

Epstein: We ourselves are not doing this population screening. The ones who are, have not defined any specific incidence of false negatives. I think it is important in these programs that those who set them up know the limits of their testing procedures, and the people who have paid most attention to this are Scriver and his collaborators in Canada, who in a sense can define the possibility of false negatives by the criteria that they use in the actual test. This is a combination of the absolute enzyme activity for hexosaminidase A and of the ratio of hexosaminidase A to total enzyme activity, and a combination of the two. Their incidence of false negatives is very low. The one group that one can run into difficulty in the screening programs is in the pregnant women in whom you get the reverse situation, the enzyme levels are altered. And in pregnant women you cannot use serum screening; you must go to screening of the white cells directly.

Edwards: I think I am right in saying that the statistical procedures used combined with the biochemical procedures are such that although they made false negatives very rare, they have only done this at the cost of making false positives very common, and I think the majority of people that are said to be heterozygotes are in fact normal homozygotes. So this is one of the problems; it seems you can only get a low number of false negatives by a high risk of false positives, and I do not think you can altogether ignore false positives and cast them aside as not being a problem.

Epstein: No, the general practice of those who screen as you describe is that the positives are then followed up by direct analysis on cells, and they no longer use the same system. I think they can eliminate the incidence of false positives in that way.

van Gemund: Are you aware of animal models, for example the mouse, or are there human cells that can be used in vitro?

Epstein: There is one mouse model with a disorder of this type, which is called foam-cell reticulosis; it was thought to be a Niemann-Pick-like disorder, but I think the enzyme defect is somewhat different. That is the one possible animal model. I think people are trying to develop *in vitro* models; we ourselves are interested in *in vitro* models using human cells. Most of the work has been done with fibroblasts, but that is not the right cell because the fibroblast usually does not store the material. Our own interest is in trying to use the macrophage as an *in vitro* model; whether it will succeed or not I do not know. Animals are much less affected with this group of disorders, at least this holds for mice, which have been screened for almost everything. I do not know whether it is just the rarity or that our ability to detect them is much poorer.

SPINA BIFIDA AND ANENCEPHALY

J. H. EDWARDS

These diverse disorders, due respectively to disturbances to the closing of the posterior and anterior neuropore, are usually regarded as central nervous system, or CNS, abnormalities, although the primary abnormality is likely to be a disorder of some common tissue with a mechanical influence on the folding of the neural crests and flexion of the embryo; the notochord is one of the best candidates, and direct observations show its remnants are often abnormal at birth (1). If this is so, the teratogens are likely to be acting on very primitive enzyme systems which will have to be studied on notochordal species or by specialized culture techniques.

These disorders are often associated in families: they are often said to be associated in individuals but this is an error perpetuated by verbal confusion between spina bifida and craniorachischisis. These primary embryological events lead to various catastrophic consequences. In anencephaly the brain is missing, there is exudation of cerebrospinal fluid which increases the amniotic fluid outflow, and the pituitary is usually small or absent. Club feet are usual.

In spina bifida the secondary effects include an increased incidence of breech delivery, dislocation of the hips, and obstruction of spinal fluid flow, leading to hydrocephalus. Isolated hydrocephalus does not coexist with spina bifida in sibships, and, excepting the rare sex-linked form (2, 3) carries an excellent prognosis for further pregnancies. This is frequently misquoted in books on counseling. Hydrocephalus in males is an indication for ultrasound but there is no indication for amniocentesis.

Both anencephaly and spina bifida are detectable by the exudation of fetal proteins into the amniotic fluid (4), and, since some proteins are only found in fetal or neural tissue, their recognition allows diagnosis in utero, provided the lesion is sufficiently severe. This provides a technical basis for the elimination of afflicted fetuses: the demand for this varies according to the survival rate at birth, which is low in some paediatric centres which do not encourage neurosurgical interference; in these areas there is no major problem which creates a demand for fetal diagnosis.

Prevention is, at present, impossible due to absence of the known teratogens, the early promise of the potato fungicides as a cause not being substantiated (5). The marked influence of numerous environmental features on incidence implies that this is largely a preventable disease, while the small size of afflicted embryos suggests a general growth impairment, which is likely to handicap numerous other fetuses who are not afflicted with any obvious abnormality.

A study of the environmental variations have clearly shown that these disorders are predisposed to by primiparity, by increased maternal age, by poor social class, by year, by season and by locality (6). Unfortunately locality is difficult to dissociate from racial background, but, even if we attribute the major differences in incidence between the Irish and the French, or even the considerable but smaller differences between the Irish and the Scots, or the East and West Coast Scots, we are dealing with fairly homogenous groups of *fetuses* whose liabilities to affliction are varying several fold. That is, if most fetuses had the risk of the low risk fetus, classified on purely environmental grounds, most cases would not occur.

Unfortunately the major factors have resisted discovery so far, and the failure to confirm the very plausible theory of Renwick (5) by any adequate protection following a potato-free pregnancy, seems to have reduced, rather than increased, the deployment of resources for prevention. In retrospect we can expect to look as foolish as our predecessors did in their slowness to appreciate the infective nature of tuberculosis, or the nutritional nature of rickets, to cite two strongly familial disorders of the past.

Once found, the avoidance of this teratogen – and, as both lung-cancer and cigarette induced neonatal weakness have shown, detection and avoidance are by no means the same – will allow preventive measures to be instituted in the true sense of the word.

Since spina bifida is associated with a degree of growth impairment which cannot be explained by the disorder itself, it is reasonable to suppose that the disorder is an extreme manifestation, and that a withdrawal of the teratogen will lead to a general improvement in fetal health.

Parents whose children have spina bifida and anencephaly have often received genetic advice, although the rationale for doing so is unclear, since the aetiology is unknown. However, where advice on recurrence is requested, the figures, which are based on many series, the most recent being that of Carter and Evans (7), show a recurrence risk of about 3% for the same defect and 2% for the other following either spina bifida or anencephaly. Some families with a considerable concentration, extending over more than one generation, are sometimes found, and in those a worse prognosis must be given. After two affected children the risks increase to about 10%. Parents are mostly concerned at the risk of a crippled child and this is about 3% in spina bifida and 2% in anencephaly. Anencephaly is, of course, a fatal condition, and, of itself, hardly presents any indication for fetal diagnosis.

A prognosis of a risk of 3% or even 5% hardly influences reproduction and, since almost all cases will be first cases, can hardly affect incidence. Treatment of cases will have a slight effect for the same reason; the risk to the children of those afflicted is increased, and is probably of the same order as sib recurrence, so that, even if treatment were invariably successful, not more than 3% of cases would have affected parents; that is, those afflicted would not increase more than 3% per year. This tendency for children to have the defects of their parents in no way implies that a reduction in the levels of teratogens would not reduce the incidence of affliction.

Since prevention is impractical, as the teratogens are unknown, and genetic counseling, even if appropriate, ineffective, the only alternative to the birth of spina bifida, with the distressing dilemma of natural death or unnatural life opened up by neurosurgical advances and antibiotics, is that of allowing death to precede birth by fetal diagnosis and abortion, a procedure best termed elimination. It certainly is not prevention.

As spina bifida is commoner than all the other severe viable disorders capable of fetal diagnosis put together, and as its consequences are even more tragic than most of these, the fetal diagnosis of spina bifida has more to offer, in terms of the evasion of family tragedy, than any other form of fetal diagnosis, for those families which consider fetal diagnosis acceptable.

The prevention of second afflicted cases is now possible from the discovery that serum proteins, which are unique to the fetus, will diffuse into the amniotic fluid through a defective skin covering; in practice such defects are restricted to spina bifida, anencephaly, and exomphalos. Spina bifida with a skin covering, which is usually mild in manifestation, will not be detected.

The test probably reduces the risk of a crippled child from about 3% to less than 1%. The procedures are now well developed (8), and sixteen weeks appears the best time. No false positives have been detected; that is, no normal fetuses have been aborted. Skin covered lesions have, of course, been missed; two of these occurred this year in the Birmingham area. The technical problems are not serious, although, until recently, reliable commercial antisera have been lacking. As there is little species variation in α-fetoprotein there is no shortage of antigen.

The pattern of familiarity has been used to estimate the heritability of these disorders; however, all that can be estimated is familiarity, and this is uninformative about the prospects of prevention by the identification of teratogens.

Amniocentesis following an affected pregnancy can do nothing to reduce the incidence of the 95% of cases which occur as the first in the family. The possibilities of inferring a leakage of fetal plasma by detecting its further diffusion from the amniotic fluid into the maternal plasma might seem remote; however, this seems possible and practical, and very promising results are being reported from Edinburgh, where the association with α-fetoprotein was discovered, from Glasgow, and from London. As yet, much of this work is unpublished. This introduced problems of organization, since the test should be integrated with other tests, such as those for blood group, syphilis and infective hepatitis which are normally routine during early pregnancy. The detection of maternal α-fetoprotein is difficult, and radio-immunoassay is necessary. If these can be delayed until the 12th-16th week, or whenever the optimal time is found to be, then all these tests can be done at the same time. It is, of course, extremely important not to allow the situation to arise in which the woman who will not permit termination is told that she is carrying a crippled child. The situation can only be avoided if the test is not done surreptitiously; that is, if women sign a document authorizing tests which might lead to a diagnosis of incurable fetal disorders.

Since spina bifida is by far the commonest fetal disease capable of elimination, being two or three times commoner than mongolism, about a hundred times commoner than Hurler's syndrome, and, even in Jewish communities, several times commoner than Tay-Sach's disease, the organization of any fetal screening must give priority to this disorder. Since the acquisition of amniotic fluid is not a safe procedure – and anyone who thinks otherwise would be well advised to desert the library for the operating theatre and watch the procedure – there is an obligation to test any fluid as exhaustively as possible. There are unfortunately economic reasons for not being able to examine all amniotic fluids taken from patients who have had spina bifida children for mongolism; however, α-fetoprotein testing is cheap, and, the protein resists freezing. Any amniotic specimen taken with a view to fetal diagnosis which is not tested for α-fetoprotein would seem to constitute a misuse of opportunity verging on malpractice.

If fetal screening is to be done then spina bifida is the disorder around which the procedure must be centralized. Not only is it more important than mongolism numerically; it causes suffering to those afflicted, and even greater distress to relatives. This is, of course, just a stop-gap procedure until the teratogens are identified, but, until then, it presents the most important indication for fetal diagnosis. It is a straightforward obstetric problem to which genetic counseling has no obvious relevance, although it has been advanced and developed almost entirely by departments of genetics.

The policy of screening all women over 40 by amniocentesis for mongolism will have a fetal mortality of over 1% from the procedure itself – the true fetal mortality is difficult to estimate but it has been estimated at 2% in one of the most experienced units; I know of two fetal deaths from haemorrhage in a series considerably smaller than a hundred. Most published series seem remarkably free from incident.

Even if the test only induces 1% of fetal deaths, this means that, since only 1% of births will be mongols, half the abortions will be of normal fetuses. In spina bifida the risks on recurrence data are 3%, and the chance that a high maternal serum α-fetoprotein will be confirmed on amniocentesis is probably higher than 3%. That is to say, the majority of terminations induced following amniocentesis for high maternal levels will be of afflicted fetuses.

REFERENCES

1. Marin-Padilla, M., Study of the sphenoid bone in human cranioschisis and cranio-rachischisis. *Virchows Arch. path. Anat. 339:* 245 (1965).
2. Bickers, D. A. and R. D. Adams, Hereditary stenosis of the aqueduct of Sylvius as a cause of congenital hydrocephalus. *Brain 72:* 246 (1949).
3. Edwards, J. H., The Syndrome of Sex-linked Hydrocephalus. *Arch. Dis. Childh. 36:* 486 (1961).
4. Brock, D. J. H. and R. G. Sutcliffe, Alpha-Fetoprotein in the Antenatal diagnosis of Anencephaly and spina bifida. *Lancet 1:* 197 (1972).
5. Renwick, J. H., Hypothesis: Anenecephaly and Spina Bifida are usually preventable by avoidance of a specific but unidentified substance present in certain potato tubers. *Brit. J. of Prev. Soc. Med. 26:* 67 (1972).
6. Edwards, J. H., Congenital malformations of the central nervous system in Scotland. *Brit. J. of Prev. Soc. Med. 12:* 115 (1958).
7. Carter, C. O. and Kathleen Evans, Spina bifida and Anencephalus in the Greater London area. *J. med. Gen. 10:* 209 (1973).
8. Allan, Lindsey D., M. A. Ferguson-Smith, Ian Donald, Elizabeth M. Sweek and A. A. M. Gibson, Amniotic fluid fetoprotein in the antenatal diagnosis of spina bifida. *Lancet ii:* 522 (1973).

DISCUSSION

PAPER OF J. H. EDWARDS

Veltkamp: There was some mention in the literature about spina bifida being a possible example of cytoplasmic inheritance.

Edwards: Yes, I suppose it obviously is a possible example, but so is every other condition. It is difficult to see how a woman can cytoplasmically convey her material to only one twin. Furthermore, it does not explain the great fluctuations, between winter and summer, and so on. It is very difficult to get split marriage data, but I think there is evidence that this condition goes through the female line more strongly than the male, but so does diet in most families.

van Rood: Are seasonal and regional differences in the birth frequency of spina bifida really significant?

Edwards: Yes, very significant differences, with variations, however, from year to year and from area to area, but there is no doubt it is a very sustained effect. It has been dropping off recently, which is difficult to understand, but of course the diet is now much less seasonal with deep-freeze, not to mention the Common Market with its mountains of beef, butter, and so on. Since 1946 there have been very reliable data from Scotland and later from other countries showing a very much weaker way, but formerly it was not actually significant. There is also a very big difference in immigrants to Australia, for example, who have a much lower incidence than expected. The assumption was that it should go the other way in Australia, but it was such a rare condition that it was not possible to collect sufficient data.

van Rood: There was a report about linkage between HLA and spina bifida.

Edwards: Yes, I am afraid I have not seen it, and I cannot quite see how you could get linkage data with this because families are so rare.

Eriksson: Do you agree with a possible influence of potatoes in the diet on the development of spina bifida?

Edwards: In Birmingham we have worked on the potato for some time, particularly Dr. Record, who is not only a good, knowledgeable epidemiologist but actually grows potatoes himself. We thought at that time of an alkaloid, because a potato is a severely toxic thing. It is obviously just waiting to be eaten by a variety of animals which are not able to tolerate it. It cannot run away and it is full of the most ferocious biological substances; if you put it just near some red cells they agglutinate almost before they touch it. It has very powerful agglutinins and it has a set of these substances, only recently described, that are toxic to fungi, which are after all quite advanced organisms. These substances are not broken down by cooking and are even volatile, and so we thought this agreed with some of the well-known toxins, which occur in the potato when it goes green. In Belfast the incidence of spina bifida is very high. They persuaded a large group of women to go on a potato-free diet, and of the first twenty of these women two gave birth to affected babies. So this was obviously not helping very much. Still, everybody was being advised not to eat the potato for this reason, and Dr. Renwick even went to the extreme of telling women not to touch potatoes, even to get their neighbours in, to peel them if their husbands insisted on having potatoes.

Dr. Renwick thinks the Belfast study only proves that whatever the toxin was, it was very stable and lasted more than nine months. But this seems rather unlikely, and I think it must be some other substance or group of substances.

PRENATAL DIAGNOSIS OF GENETIC DISEASE

H. GALJAARD, E. S. SACHS, W. J. KLEIJER AND M. F. NIERMEIJER

INTRODUCTION

Of all newborns, 4-6% show a more or less severe congenital abnormality (1). In the Netherlands this means that annually 8.000-12.000 handicapped children are born. About 2.000 of these are affected with a genetic disease caused by a single gene mutation in the parental germ cells. At the moment nearly two thousand different traits of Mendelian inheritance are known in man (2) and in about 10% of these the biochemical lesion has been characterized (3).

Only in very few of these metabolic diseases can severe physical and mental handicaps be prevented by therapeutic measures. Also it is not to be expected that gene mutations will be prevented in the future. As a consequence parents at risk for a genetic disease are confronted with the difficult choice of either accepting a high risk (usually 1 in 4) of having a handicapped child or giving up the possibility of extending their family with healthy children. The society as a whole is faced with the heavy responsibility for optimal medical and social care of the large number of handicapped people. At the same time facilities are required for the search of new means of prevention and therapy of serious handicaps. Since in the Western European countries an increasing proportion of infant morbidity (about 25%) is due to congenital diseases more and more attention is being given to *early diagnosis of genetic diseases and to the genetic counseling* of the parents at risk.

The possibility of *prenatal diagnosis of certain genetic diseases* has opened new perspectives in genetic counseling because parents at risk can now avoid the birth of a seriously affected child by selective abortion if an abnormality is detected early in pregnancy. Moreover, the possibility of prenatal monitoring will encourage certain couples to extend their family which they would otherwise not have dared to because of a high genetic risk.

While prenatal monitoring is promising as yet several problems are involved. For a reliable analysis of the chromosome pattern or of biochemical defects in the fetus, a collaboration of investigators in different fields is required.

Usually the clinicians, geneticists, cell biologists and biochemists are very much involved in their own work, have their own methodology and think in their own terms. Sometimes this makes communication difficult and the danger exists that the patient or the parents may feel lost. In prenatal diagnosis it is not sufficient to obtain reliable analytical data but the results should also be discussed correctly with the parents and they should be helped to accept the consequences of prenatal diagnosis.

Some of the results and experiences obtained in a series of about 300 prenatal diagnoses in our centre at the Rotterdam Medical Faculty will be described.

METHODOLOGY OF PRENATAL DIAGNOSIS

The cells in amniotic fluid are mostly derived from fetal skin and mucous membranes; their number increases during gestation but the percentage of viable cells decreases. Various groups have established that the optimal period for amniocentesis is between the 14th and 16th week of pregnancy (4). In earlier gestational stages the amount of amniotic fluid present is too small, the puncture is more difficult and the in vitro growth of the relatively few viable amniotic fluid cells is too slow. After ultrasonographic localisation of the placenta and fetus, 10-15 ml of amniotic fluid is obtained via transabdominal amniocentesis under local anesthesia. This procedure gives no maternal complications and the risk for the fetus is considered to be low i.e. in the order of 1% (4, 5). To avoid gross contamination with maternal blood cells the first few milliliters of fluid are discarded. Plastic syringes or siliconized tubes are to be preferred to prevent loss of viable fetal cells. Amniotic fluid samples can be transported or kept at room temperature for a few days, and methods have been developed to store the samples with maintenance of the viability of the fetal cells (6).

After centrifugation the amniotic fluid supernatant can be used for the α-fetoprotein analysis to investigate whether or not the fetus is affected with an open defect of the neural tube (spina bifida cystica or anencephaly) (7).

The cell pellet can be cultured under special conditions (4) and various methods have been successfully used to obtain sufficient dividing cells for a chromosome preparation within 10-20 days after amniocentesis. The general opinion is that experience with (amniotic fluid) cell cultivation techniques is more important than the particular procedure used. Accurate karyotyping of the fetus requires that the amniotic fluid cells are grown in more than one culture dish and that the prepaıations are stained with one of the more recently developed staining techniques for chromosome identification (8).

In order to monitor for X-linked diseases fetal sex can be determined by staining with the fluorescent dye atebrin which shows the presence of Y-chromatin or inactivated X-chromatin in interphase nuclei (9). Although a rapid answer about fetal sex can be obtained by using this technique on uncultured amniotic fluid cells, most investigators agree that a 100% reliability can only be obtained if cells are cultivated and a complete karyotype is made (4, 10).

For the biochemical assay of enzyme deficiencies or of specific metabolites amniotic fluid cell cultivation has to be continued until sufficient cell material is available to assay the protein content, the activity of the enzyme involved in the particular metabolic disease and preferably that of a reference enzyme. Rather long cultivation periods (4-8 weeks) are required when conventional biochemical techniques are used (4, 11, 12). Such a long waiting period is of psychological disadvantage for the parents and an interruption of the pregnancy in the case of an affected fetus, is more complicated.

Microtechniques which were originally developed for the analysis of microdissected parts of tissue sections (14, 15) can be successfully used to accelerate prenatal diagnosis of some metabolic disorders (13, 16, 17). Amniotic fluid cells are cultivated on small petri dishes with a thin plastic bottom and after a few cell clones have developed in 8-14 days the dish is quickly frozen and freeze-dried in vacuum at low temperature. Counted groups of lyophilized cells (100-300 cells) can then be dissected under the microscope together with the piece of plastic on which they have grown. These cells are then incubated in (sub)microliter droplets of substrate in small wells drilled in a teflon plate; incubation is carried out under paraffin oil to prevent evaporation. The fluorescent or coloured product formed during the chemical reaction can be measured in small glass capillaries using a microscope spectrofluorometer. The enzyme activities are then expressed per cell. The various steps of this procedure are ilustrated in figure 1.

The results of the assays on cultured amniotic fluid cells should be compared with those on cells of a control amniotic fluid sample from the same gestation period and cultured under similar conditions. Furthermore biochemical data are required from cultured skin fibroblasts derived from a patient and from heterozygous carriers from the family concerned. Cell

METHODS FOR MICROCHEMICAL ANALYSES OF SMALL NUMBERS OF FREEZE-DRIED CELLS

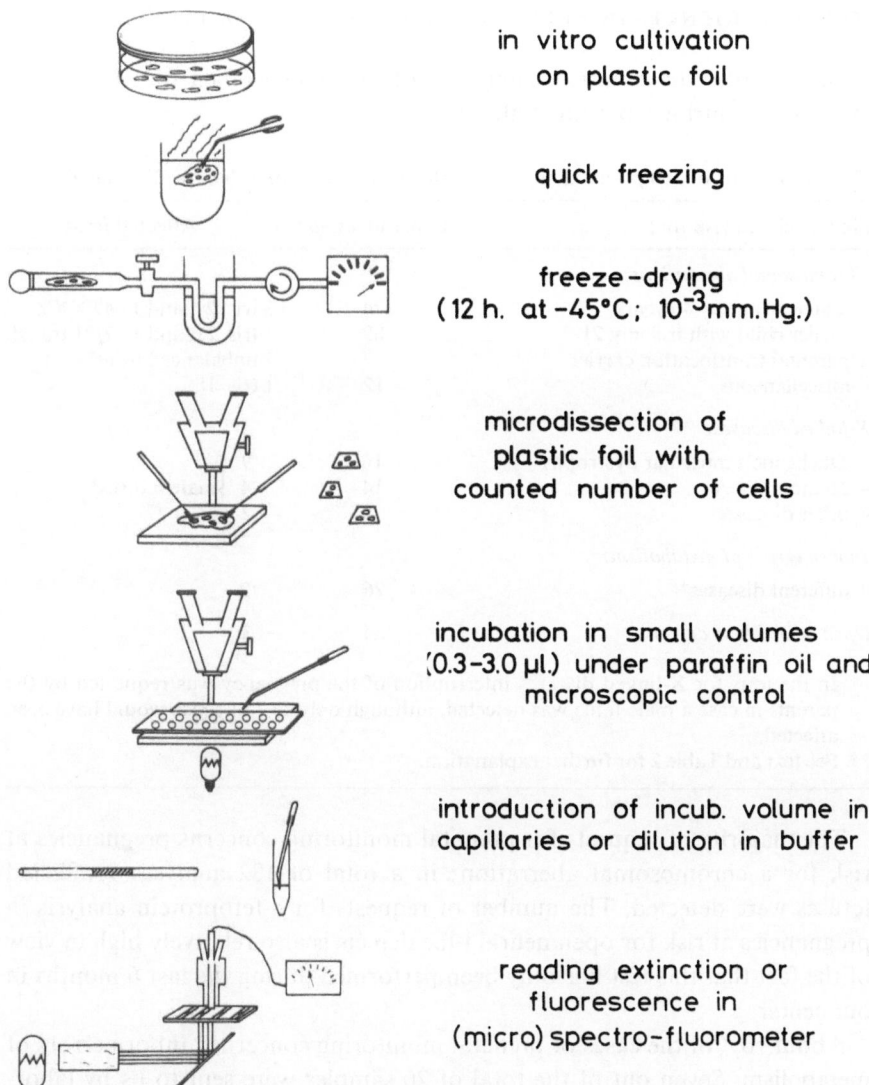

in vitro cultivation
on plastic foil

quick freezing

freeze-drying
(12 h. at -45°C; 10^{-3} mm.Hg.)

microdissection of
plastic foil with
counted number of cells

incubation in small volumes
(0.3–3.0 µl.) under paraffin oil and
microscopic control

introduction of incub. volume in
capillaries or dilution in buffer

reading extinction or
fluorescence in
(micro) spectro-fluorometer

Fig. 1. Procedure of microchemical assay on small numbers of cultured amniotic fluid cells for prenatal diagnosis of metabolic diseases.

cultivation has to be carried out under standardized conditions since the activity of several enzymes involved in genetic diseases may vary considerably under different cell cultivation conditions (4, 18, 19, 20).

SOME EXPERIENCES IN APPLICATION OF PRENATAL ANALYSIS

Table 1 shows the different categories of pregnant women that have been investigated during a period of about two years.

Table 1. Results of 280 prenatal analyses performed at the Rotterdam medical faculty.

Pregnancies at risk for:	Number investigated	Affected fetus
Chromosomal aberrations:		
– maternal age > 40 years	74	3 tris. 21, and 1 47 XXY
– earlier child with trisomy 21	89	1 tris. 21, and 1 7/21 transl.
– parental translocation carrier	7	2 unbalanced transl.
– miscellaneous	12	1 tris. 18
X-linked diseases:		
– Duchenne's muscular dystrophy	16	9
– Hemophilia A	14	4 male fetuses*
– other diseases	8	2
Inborn errors of metabolism:		
9 different diseases**	26	2
Open neural tube defects:	34	3

* In the tests for X-linked diseases interruption of the pregnancy was requested by the parents in case a male fetus was detected, although only 1:2 of those would have been affected.
** See text and Table 2 for further explanation.

The majority of requests for prenatal monitoring concerns pregnancies at risk for a chromosomal aberration: in a total of 182 analyses 9 affected fetuses were detected. The number of requests for α-fetoprotein analysis in pregnancies at risk for open neural tube defects is also relatively high in view of the fact that this test has only been performed during the last 6 months in our center.

About 10% of the cases of prenatal monitoring concerned inborn errors of metabolism. Seven out of the total of 26 samples were sent to us by laboratories from other countries. In all instances prenatal monitoring was carried out because of the occurrence of one or more affected children in the family.

(Micro)biochemical assays for nine different metabolic disorders were performed on cultured amniotic fluid cells as listed in Table 2. Only on two

Table 2. Prenatal diagnosis of inborn errors of metabolism.

Indication	Number of Pregnancies	Type of assay	Cell cultivation period
Glycogenosis II	12	1 µl cell homogenate or freeze-dried cell groups in 1-2 µl 4MU glucopyranoside pH 4.5	10-20 days
Fabry's disease	1	freeze-dried cell groups in 0.3-0.6 µl, 4 MU α-galactopyranoside pH 4.0.	10
GM1-Gangliosidosis	2	1 µl cell homogenate or freeze-dried cells in 0.3-2 µl 4 MU β-galactopyranoside pH 4.2	8-15
GM2-Gangliosidosis Tay-Sachs	3	1 µl cell homogenate or freeze-dried cells in 0.3-2 µl 4MU deoxy-β-Dglucopyranoside either or not after 2 hr. 50°C	13-15
GM2-Gangliosidosis Sandhoff	1	idem without heat inactivation	*
Metachromatic leuco-dystrophy	2	0.1 µl cell homogenate in 0.5-5 µl p. nitrocatechol sulphate pH 5.0	16-19
Mucopolysaccharidosis Hunter	3	$S^{35}O_4$ incorporation and chase studies	14
Mucopolysaccharidosis Hurler	1	idem + α-L. iduronidase assay	23
Maple syrup urine disease	1	C^{14} leucine decarboxylation in microvolumes	11

* cultivated cells obtained from elsewhere.

occasions (for glycogenosis II or Pompe's disease) was an affected fetus detected and the diagnosis confirmed by enzyme assays in fetal tissues after interruption of the pregnancy.

In one prenatal analysis for Pompe's disease a very low activity of acid α-1.4-glucosidase in cultured amniotic fluid cells from the pregnancy at risk was misinterpreted. The pregnancy was interrupted because the enzyme activity found was five times lower than that in control amniotic fluid cells. Furthermore the activity was only 2-4 times higher than that in different fibroblast strains from patients with Pompe's disease and one third of the lowest value observed in fibroblasts from heterozygous carriers. However, assays on fetal tissues could not confirm the prenatal diagnosis. Later it was found that the activity of acid α-glucosidase increases during prolonged growth after subculture of control amniotic fluid cells (18) and the misinterpretation could be explained by the fact that in this particular prenatal diagnosis control amniotic fluid cells from a later passage had been used instead of primary cultures. All subsequent analytical results of cultured cells from pregnancies at risk were compared with those of primary cultures of control amniotic fluid cells grown at the same time. The necessity of using control cells grown under comparable conditions probably applies to the prenatal diagnosis of many other metabolic diseases since it has been shown that the activity of several enzymes increases during the growth curve in later subcultures of amniotic fluid cells as well as in skin fibroblasts (4, 18, 19, 20). The use of primary cultures as controls is especially important in early prenatal diagnosis using microtechniques as this enables biochemical analysis of the few cells which are already available after 10-14 days in primary culture (16, 21). Primary cultures of normal amniotic fluid may be obtained at any desired time because uncultured amniotic fluid samples can be stored in liquid nitrogen with maintenance of cell viability (6).

Another prerequisite in prenatal diagnosis is that skin fibroblasts should be available from an affected patient and heterozygous carriers of the same family which requests amniocentesis. In an increasing number of metabolic disorders the residual enzyme activity is seen to vary between patients from different families (4, 18, 26). In addition to differences arising from cell cultivation conditions these variations may be due to genetic factors. In Table 3 such variations are illustrated for a number of lysosomal enzymes in

Table 3. Variations in (residual) enzyme activity in cultured fibroblasts from different individuals.

	Acid α-1.4-glucosidase*			Arylsulphatase A**			Hexosaminidase ratio A:B***		
Controls	473,	1010,	3280,	7.6,	10.0,	8.2,	1.0,	1.4,	1.0,
	2760,	1920,	1780	10.8,	5.2		1.1,	0.9,	0.6
Heterozygotes	1654,	352,	475,	4.2,	3.4,	3.7,	0.6,	2.1,	1.2,
	351,	480,	310	2.2,	5.3,	2.7	2.1,	2.4	
Affected patients	59,	21,	25,	0.2,	0.1,	0.0,	0.16,	0.15,	0.45,
	27,	22,	28	0.4,	0.0		0.20		

* Assays performed in methylumbelliferyl glucopyranoside pH 4.5 and activities expressed × 10⁻¹² mole/min/mg protein.** p.nitrocatechol sulphate, pH 5.0 and activities expressed × 10⁻⁹ mole/min/mg protein. *** for total hexos. activity 1 hour incubation in methylumbelliferyl substrate pH 4.4 and for hex. A incubation after inactivation 2 hours at 50°C.

skin fibroblasts from controls, heterozygous carriers and from different patients with the same metabolic disease. For a reliable prenatal diagnosis it is required that the metabolic disease in that particular family has been diagnosed by the demonstration of the biochemical defect in leucocytes, tissue biopsies or cultured skin fibroblasts. Furthermore fibroblasts of an affected sibling should be stored in a cell bank until required for future prenatal diagnosis. Clinicians should be warned to take such skin biopsies in good time.

The genetic background of variations in residual enzyme activity in patients with seemingly identical metabolic diseases and that of the heterogeneity in clinical and pathological manifestations can be investigated by somatic cell hybridization techniques. For a few inborn errors of metabolism it has been shown that different clinical and/or biochemical variants are caused by different gene mutations since enzyme activity is restored after fusion of enzyme deficient cell strains derived from two different patients (22, 23, 24). Such genetic complementation studies are complicated by the fact that no selection method exists for the isolation of hybrid cells. The microtechniques described earlier in this paper permit quantitation of enzymes on single cultured cells (16), which enables genetic complementation studies on individual binuclear hybrid cells.

The application of such methods has already contributed to the genetic classification of different clinical and biochemical variants of the lysosomal storage disease GM1-gangliosidosis (25). It is to be expected that in the near future such hybridization studies will provide more information about the genetic heterogeneity existing in several metabolic disorders (3). Such information might also be useful in the genetic counseling and prenatal diagnosis of inborn errors of metabolism.

The reliability of (prenatal) diagnosis of metabolic diseases will improve if the necessary analyses are performed in centres which have acquired sufficient experience in biochemical and genetic aspects of the diseases concerned and also in the interpretation of analytical data in relation to cell cultivation conditions. Such experience can only be accumulated when analyses for the (prenatal) diagnosis of relatively rare metabolic diseases are concentrated in few specialized centres. Only close collaboration between clinicians, biochemists, cell-biologists and geneticists will enable the translation of laboratory results into the maximum benefit to parents at risk.

REFERENCES

1. Warkany, J., *Congenital malformations*. Year Book Medical Publ. Inc. Chicago 1971.
2. McKusick, V. A., *Mendelian inheritance in man*. 3rd ed. John Hopkins, Baltimore 1971.
3. Stanbury, J. B., J. B. Wijngaarden and D. S. Fredrickson, *The metabolic basis of inherited disease*. 3rd ed. Mc.Graw Hill, New York 1972.
4. Milunsky, A., *The prenatal diagnosis of hereditary disorders*. C. Thomas Publ., Springfield 1973.
5. Fuchs, F., In: *Intrauterine diagnosis*. Birth Defects Series. Vol. VII, No. 5, p. 18, April 1971.
6. Niermeijer, M. F., D. Halley, E. S. Sachs, C. Tichelaar-Klepper and K. Garver, Transport and storage of amniotic fluid samples for prenatal diagnosis of metabolic diseases. *Humangenetik 20:* 175, 1973.
7. Brock, D. H. J. and R. G. Sutcliffe, Alpha-fetoprotein in the antenatal diagnosis of anencephaly and spina bifida. *Lancet* ii: 197, 1972.
8. Paris Conference on Standardization in human cytogenetics. *Cytogenetics 11:* 313, 1971.
9. Pearson, P. L., M. Bobrow and C. G. Vosa, *Nature 226:* 78, 1970.
10. McIntyre, M. N., In: *Intrauterine diagnosis*. Birth Defects Series. Original Article Series. Vol. VII, no. 5, p. 10, April 1971.
11. Nadler, H. L., Tissue culture and antenatal detection of molecular diseases. *Biochimie 54:* 677, 1972a.
12. Nadler, H. L., In: *Advances in Human Genetics* 3. pp. 1-38. H. Harris and K. Hirschhorn, (eds.). Plenum Press, New York 1972b.
13. Galjaard, H., J. J. van Hoogstraten, J. E. de Josselin de Jong and M. P. Mulder, Methodology of quantitative cytochemical analysis of single or small numbers of cultured cells. *Histochem. J. 6:* 409, 1974.
14. Lowry, O. H. and J. V. Passonneau, *A flexible system of enzyme analysis*. Acad. Press, New York 1972.
15. Dubach, U. C. and U. Schmidt, Recent advances in Quantitative Histo- and Cytochemistry, *Huber Publ.* Bern 1971.
16. Galjaard, H., A. Hoogeveen, W. Keijzer, H. A. de Wit-Verbeek and C. Vlek-Noot, The use of quantitative cytochemical analyses in rapid prenatal detection and somatic cell genetic studies of metabolic diseases. *Histochem. J. 6:* 491, 1974.
17. Galjaard, H., M. Mekes, J. E. de Josselin de Jong and M. F. Niermeijer, A method for rapid prenatal diagnosis of glycogenosis II. *Clin. Chim. Acta 49:* 361, 1973.
18. Galjaard, H., A. J. J. Reuser, M. J. Heukels-Dully, A. Hoogeveen, W. Keijzer, H. A. de Wit-Verbeek and M. F. Niermeijer, In: *Enzyme therapy in lysosomal storage diseases*. J. Tager, G. J. M. Hooghwinkel and W. Th. Daems, (eds.). p. 35, North Holland Publ. Cy., Amsterdam 1974.
19. Milunsky, A., C. Spielvogel and J. N. Kanfer, Lysosomal enzyme variations in cultured normal skin fibroblasts. *Life Sci. 11:* 1101, 1972.
20. Sutherland, G. R., J. Butterworth, D. M. Broadhead and D. M. Bain, Lysosomal enzyme levels in human amniotic fluid cells in tissue culture. *Clin. Genet. 5:* 351, 1974.
21. Galjaard, H., M. F. Niermeijer, N. Hahnemann, J. Mohr and S. A. Sørensen, An example of rapid prenatal diagnosis of Fabry's disease using microtechniques. *Clin. Genet. 5:* 368, 1974.
22. Weerd-Kastelein, E. A. de, W. Keijzer and D. Bootsma, Genetic heterogeneity of Xeroderma pigmentosum demonstrated by somatic cell hybridization. *Nature New Biol. 238:* 80, 1972.
23. Thomas, G. H., H. A. Taylor, C. S. Miller, J. Axelman and B. R. Migeon, Genetic

complementation after fusion of Tay-Sachs and Sandhoff cells. *Nature New Biology* *250:* 580, 1974.
24. Galjaard, H., A. Hoogeveen, H. A. de Wit-Verbeek, A. J. J. Reuser, W. Keijzer, A. Westerveld and D. Bootsma, Tay-Sachs and Sandhoff's disease: Intergenic complementation after somatic cell hybridization. *Exptl. Cell Res. 87:* 444, 1974.
25. Galjaard, H., A. Hoogeveen, W. Keijzer, H. A. de Wit-Verbeek and A. J. J. Reuser, *Different Gene mutations in variants of GM1- and GM2-gangliosidosis demonstrated by enzyme analysis of (single) somatic hybrid cells.* In: Rotterdam Conference 1974. Second International Workshop on human Gene mapping, p. 150 (The National Foundation, New York 1975).
26. Kaback, M., C. O. Leonard and T. H. Parmiley, Intrauterine diagnosis: comparative enzymology of cells cultivated from maternal skin, fetal skin and amniotic fluid cells. *Pediat. Res. 5:* 366, 1971.

DISCUSSION

PAPER OF H. GALJAARD C.S.

Tan: How do you get normal amnion cells for control?

Galjaard: At present, the medical centres working on prenatal diagnosis of spina bifida and anencephaly get a lot of amniotic fluid in the period between 12 and 16 weeks. We need only the supernatant of the amniotic fluid for the determination of spina bifida and of alpha-fetoprotein, so we can use these cells as controls.

Anders: I suppose that this solution for getting cells will not last very long because the serum of the mother is being increasingly used for the alpha-fetoprotein determination.

Galjaard: In the break I discussed this matter with Dr. Edwards, and he is of the opinion that this determination is not reliable as yet.

DETECTION OF CARRIERS OF HEMOPHILIA

J. J. VELTKAMP, E. BRIËT, M. M. VAN DER KLAUW AND
J. M. H. HERMANS

INTRODUCTION

Hemophilia is the general name for sexlinked inherited bleeding disorders, apparently well-known in the ancient Jewish and Arabic literature (1), as can be inferred from regulations for dispensation from circumcision. Dispensation was granted when maternal uncles had shown overt bleeding or even died from bleeding after circumcision.

In 1935 Haldane concluded from Davenport's data that the disease was heterogeneous, probably due to a series of allelomorphic genes explaining for differences in clinical severity within families. In 1952 a major distinction was made (2) in hemophilia A and B, being completely different biochemically but both showing sex-linked inheritance and also variable clinical severity between families. Since then it was possible to assay the activity of the coagulation factor VIII, absent or diminished in hemophilia A (classic hemophilia) and IX, absent or diminished in hemophilia B (Christmas disease, PTC deficiency). Haldane's hypothesis, that allelomorphic genes exist, was confirmed on basis of the correlation of factor VIII activity levels of hemophiliacs within families (3, 4). Clinically the hemophilia's are classified as severe ($<$ 1% of the coagulation factor), moderately severe (1-5%), and mild (5-25%) but many more allelomorphic genes must exist.

It has never been clear whether the proteins of the clotting factor are synthetized at a slower rate or whether molecular variants are produced at a normal rate but displaying absent or lower coagulation activity. The first speculations were that both situations are in existence; about 5 percent of severely affected patients with classic hemophilia produce an inhibitor of the clotting factor activity upon transfusion with material containing human factor VIII. This inhibitor is an IgG-immunoglobulin. It was thought that those patients would not synthesize the clotting factor protein (CRM-negative) and that the remaining 95 percent of the patients would be CRM-positive. By means of such an antibody a so-called inhibitor neutralization assay was set up. It appeared that only in 5 to 10 percent of the cases the plasma of severely affected hemophiliacs could neutralize the antibody, instead of the expected 95 to 90 percent (5).

In another study (6) it is emphasized that the proportion of CRM-positive patients might differ dependent on the inhibitor used and furthermore that CRM-levels appear to be quite similar in related hemophiliacs.

In 1970 Zimmerman et al. (7) produced a precipitating antibody in rabbits against human factor VIII. With this antibody all hemophiliacs appeared to have CRM at an even slightly higher level than normals. This CRM is called AHF-related or factor VIII-like antigen.

At present all the experimental evidence is clearly demonstrating that what we call factor VIII-like antigen is in fact the von Willebrand's disease antigen. The factor VIII-like antigen is lacking or diminished in von Willebrand patients (7), the antigen has a different T50 than factor VIII activity in von Willebrand patients (8, 9), fractions with posttransfusional factor VIII activity in von Willebrand patients do not contain the antigen (10) and human 'purified' factor VIII can be separated into activity and antigen (11). The relationship between factor VIII-like antigen (von Willebrand's disease antigen) and factor VIII activity, on basis of experimental and genetic data, is limited to:

1. Both entities are found together, probably in a complexed form, in 'purified' human factor VIII; they might also circulate together as a complexed molecule.
2. The antigen, most likely the primary gene-product of the autosomal von Willebrand locus, exerts an influence (regulation, induction) on the production of factor VIII activity by an X-chromosomal locus.

Recently Zimmerman and Edgington (12) demonstrated antigenic material related to factor VIII in normal plasma present in reduced amounts in hemophilic plasma. Factor VIII is absorbable on agarose beads coated with heterologous antiserum against factor VIII, so-called 'antibody beads'. Hemophilic plasma is able to displace competitively normal factor VIII from these immobilized antibodies. Such material, probably defective factor VIII, is not present in von Willebrand plasma. This solid-phase antigen assay seems to be the most promising method for demonstrating X-chromosomal factor VIII, normal as wel as structurally altered.

For hemophilia B the situation at present is the following:

1. About 20 percent of kindreds are CRM-positive with an inhibitor-neutralization assay (13); the inhibitor used is a spontaneously occurring antibody in a patient with severe hemophilia B (14).
2. About 10 percent of patients with hemophilia B have prolonged prothrombin times with ox-brain thromboplastin. This phenomenon, thought to be caused by some kind of abnormal factor IX molecule, was named hemophilia Bm, the m being the first letter of the patient's surname (15). Plasma from hemophilia Bm patients can have inhibitor-neutralizing properties (CRM-positive) but this does not appear to be a rule (16).
3. A factor IX neutralizing antibody produced in rabbits (17) demonstrates the presence of CRM in the majority (> 90 per cent) of hemophilia B kindreds. Two investigators (18; 19) find a much lower incidence of CRM-positivity.
4. A precipitating antibody against factor IX produced in rabbits shows CRM in 90 percent of hemophilia B kindreds (20).

CARRIER DETECTION ON BASIS OF COAGULATION FACTOR LEVELS

Andreassen (21), in the era that specific clotting factor assays were not possible, found that a few carriers of hemophilia showed long whole blood clotting times. When later factor VIII and IX assays were carried out it was found that carriers show on the average 50 percent of the normal clotting factor activity. The range of levels, however, is much larger than for normals. Some obligatory carriers have very low levels, classifying them even as severely affected hemophiliacs (22), others display the highest normal levels.

Frota-Pessao (23) was the first to apply the Lyon hypothesis (24) to this phenomenon. Random inactivation of one X-chromosome in the female cell during embryonic development cannot only explain dosage compensation in the female for X-governed enzyme levels but also the wide range of clotting factor levels in the hemophilia carrier. If by chance the majority of X-chromosomes bearing the hemophilia gene are being inactivated the carrier will show a normal clotting factor level and the reverse is true when most of the normal X-chromosomes are inactivated.

In our hands detection of carriers on basis of coagulation factor levels for hemophilia A is possible in some 30 percent and for hemophilia B in 40 percent of the potential carrier population, i.e. in women with a 50 percent genetic chance of being a carrier (25). Exclusion of carriership with this method is only possible in a few percent of the cases.

Other workers (26, 27) claim to be more successful.

CARRIER DETECTION USING BOTH COAGULATION FACTOR ACTIVITY AND CRM

In this section we will only discuss detection of carriers for hemophilia A. Studies on carrier detection for hemophilia B are underway and results are not yet available.

If we could measure the level of antigen produced by the factor VIII locus on the X-chromosome, and if hemophilia A is indeed due to a structural mutation, the detection rate of carriers would be very high. In normals then we would expect identical levels of the activity and the antigen and in carriers excess of antigen over activity which would be diagnostic. In that situation only two facts are important:

1. The error in assaying factor VIII activity and antigen levels.
2. the frequency of carriers that are completely or nearly completely Lyonized into the normal direction; in other words carriers who have inactivated hemophilic X-chromosomes in all their factor VIII producing cells.

The most promising assay up to date to measure defective factor VIII (11), however, demonstrates a reduced antigenic expression in hemophiliacs. Data on carriers of classic hemophilia with this method are not yet available, but as the margin between factor VIII activity and the total amount of factor VIII, normal and defective, as measured with the solid-phase antigen assay looks theoretically very narrow, improvement of carrier detection is not to be expected.

Therefore carrier detection on the moment is based on the assay of factor VIII activity and the von Willebrand's disease antigen (factor VIII-like antigen). This approach is completely empirical, due to the obscurity of the relationship between the two entities as pointed out before.

The results of carrier detection studies of this type can be seen in Table 1. From that material which is for the most part not yet published it is evident that the optimistic attitude induced by the early results is not warranted. This is also evident from a reaction (28) on an editorial in the Lancet (29).

The separation of the normal and carrier group with both assays simultaneously, i.e. von Willebrand's disease antigen and factor VIII activity, succeeds better than with the activity assay alone. We investigated a sample of obligatory carriers (n = 20) and a sample of normals (n = 33). For each sample three tolerance ellipses were constructed, which are expected to cover respectively 50, 90, and 95% of the combination of values of factor VIII-like antigen and activity (Fig. 1). For this construction we used eq. (3.11) from Guttman (34). We found 17 normals (52 percent) to be outside

Table 1. Results of hemophilia carrier studies.

First author	Normals (n)	Obligatory carriers (n)	Percentage of carriers outside the region of the normals	Percentage of normals inside the region of the normals
Zimmerman (7)	22	25	92	99[c]
Bennett (8)	38	42	95	99[c]
Ekert (30)	20	13	77	?
Denson (31)	18	18	66[a]	?
Meyer (32)	30	49	72-82[b]	95
Prentice (28)	?	24	60	> 75[d]
Bouma (33)	30	22	82	95[e]
Present investigation	30	21	70	95[e]

a = estimated from figure.
b = dependent on statistical methods.
c = in confidence regions based on regression analysis.
d = betting odds 1 to 4 or greater.
e = tolerance regions (see text).

the 95% tolerance region of the carriers and 14 carriers (70 percent) to be outside the 95% tolerance region for normals.

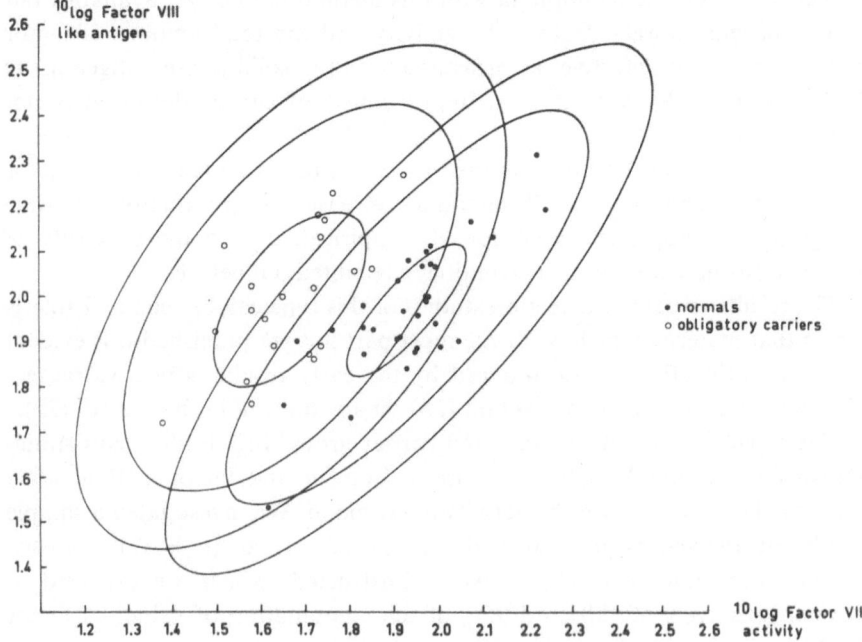

Fig. 1. Tolerance ellipses for the normal and obligatory carrier group (see text).

A woman without hemophilic relatives has a certain chance on carriership: 30 percent of all cases of hemophilia are sporadic, i.e. due to a new mutation. Females have twice the chance to receive X-chromosomal mutations as compared to males; this means that $2 \times 0.0001 \times 0.30$ (in which 2 is the double chance to receive the mutation, 0.0001 the incidence of the disease in males, and 0.30 the relative frequency of sporadic hemophilia), i.e. 0.00006 is the genetic probability (g) for a woman without hemophilic relatives to carry the hemophilia gene.

The daughter of an obligatory carrier has a genetic chance of $g = 0.5$ and it must be clear that a combination of values of factor VIII-like antigen and factor VIII activity that yields a point just outside the 95 percent tolerance region for normals enlarges her probability of being a true carrier to more than 99 percent whereas the woman with a $g = 0.00006$ and identical laboratory data still has a fair chance of being normal.

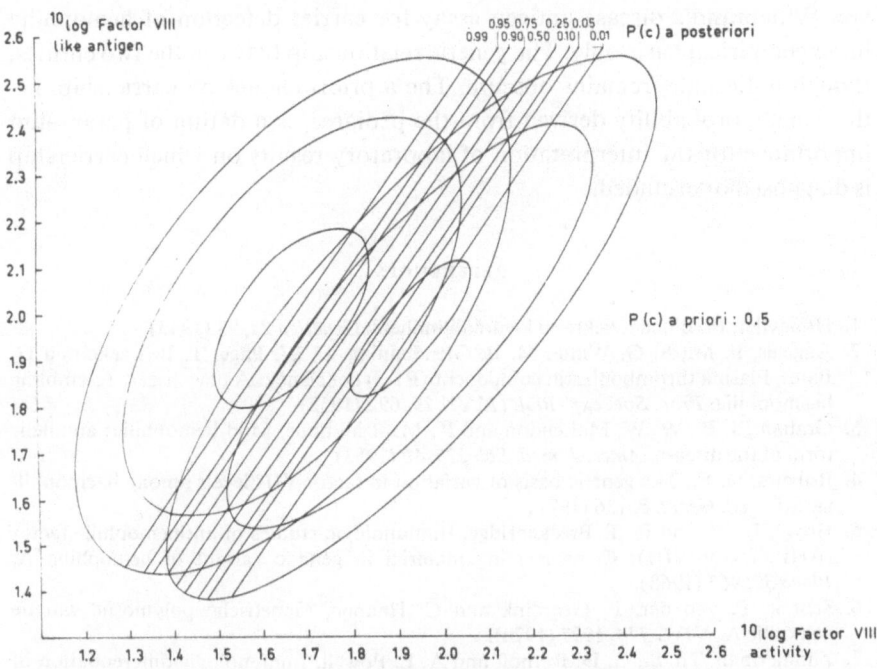

Fig. 2. Application of Bayes rule for carrier diagnosis. The probability a posteriori on carriership, in this example for a $g = 0.5$, can be read on the nomogram after plotting of the laboratory data.

For this probalistic calculation the theorem of Bayes is very suitable. For each level of genetic chance on carriership (g) the probability a posteriori can be calculated after the laboratory data are available, i.e. with known values for u and v. This theorem leads to the following expression of the probability a posteriori on carriership:

$$P(c) = \frac{g}{g + (1 - g) \exp (t(u, v))}$$

Where u = ^{10}log factor VIII activity, v = ^{10}log factor VIII-like antigen (von Willebrand's disease antigen), and t(u, v) = 32.580 u − 22.686 v + 6.138, in which t(u, v) is Fisher's linear discriminant function, and g the prior (i.e. genetically determined) probability on carriership. For the most common g's nomograms can be constructed to read the probability a posteriori (fig. 2).

In conclusion: the use of the combined data from factor VIII activity and von Willebrand's disease antigen assay for carrier detection of hemophilia has an empirical basis only. The genetic relationship between the two entities, though noticeable, remains obscure. The a priori chance on carriership, i.e. the genetic probability derived from the pedigree, is a datum of paramount importance for the interpretation of laboratory results on which carriership is diagnosed or excluded.

REFERENCES

1. Hoogvliet, B., Bloederziekte en kleurenblindheid. *Genetica 23*, 93 (1943).
2. Aggeler, P. M., S. G. White, M. B. Glendenning, E. W. Page, T. B. Laeke and G. Bates, Plasma thromboplastin component (PTC) deficiency: A new disease resembling haemophilia. *Proc. Soc. exp. Biol. (N.Y.) 79*, 692 (1952).
3. Graham, J. B., W. W. McLendon and K. M. Brinkhous, Mild hemophilia: an allelic form of the disease. *Amer. J. med. Sci. 225*, 46 (1953).
4. Roberts, D. F., The genetic basis of variation in factor VIII levels among haemophiliacs. *J. med. Genet. 8*, 136 (1971).
5. Hoyer, L. W. and R. T. Breckenridge, Immunologic studies of antihemophilic factor (AHF, factor VIII): Cross reacting material in genetic variant of hemophilia A. *Blood 32*, 962 (1968).
6. Schoot, P. van der, P. Geerdink and C. Haanen, Genetische polymorfie van de hemofilie A. *NTvG 114*, 1997 (1970).
7. Zimmerman, Th. S., O. D. Ratnoff and A. E. Powell, Immunologic differentiation of classic hemophilia (factor VIII deficiency) and von Willebrand's disease, with observations on combined deficiencies of antihemophilic factor and proaccelerin (factor V) and on an acquired circulating anticoagulant against antihemophilic factor. *J. Clin. Invest. 50*, 244 (1971).

8. Bennett, B., O. D. Ratnoff and J. Levin, Immunologic studies in von Willebrand's disease: evidence that the antihemophilic factor (AHF) produced after transfusions lacks an antigen associated with normal AHF and the inactive material produced by patients with classic hemophilia. *J. clin. Invest. 51*, 2597 (1972).
9. Veltkamp, J. J. and N. H. van Tilburg, 'Autosomal haemophilia: A variant of von Willebrand's disease. *Brit. J. Haemat. 26*, 141 (1974).
10. Bloom, A. L., J. C. Giddings and I. R. Peake, Low-molecular-weight factor VIII. *Lancet I*, 661 (1973).
11. Zimmerman, Th. S. and Th. S. Edgington, Factor VIII coagulant activity and factor VIII-like antigen: Independent molecular entities. *J. exp. Med. 138*, 1015 (1973).
12. Zimmerman, Th. S. and Th. S. Edgington, Molecular immunology of factor VIII. *Ann. Rev. Med. 25*, 303 (1974).
13. Roberts, H. R., J. E. Grizzle, W. D. McLester and G. D. Penick, Genetic variants of hemophilia B: Detection by means of a specific PTC inhibitor. *J. clin. Invest. 47*, 360 (1968).
14. Fantal, P., R. J. Sawers and A. G. Marr, Investigation of a haemorrhagic disease due to betaprothromboplastin deficiency complicated by a specific inhibitor of thromboplastin formation. *Australasian Ann. Med. 5*, 163 (1956).
15. Hougie, C. and J. J. Twomey, Haemophilia Bm: A new type of factor-IX deficiency. *Lancet I*, 698 (1967).
16. Meyer, D., M. J. Larrieu and B. Obert, Factor VIII and IX variants. Relationship between haemophilia Bm and haemophilia B+. *Europ. J. clin. Invest. I*, 425 (1971).
17. Meyer, D., E. Bidwell and M. J. Larrieu, Cross reacting material in genetic variants of haemophilia B. *J. clin. Path. 25*, 433 (1972).
18. Elödi, S. and E. Puskas, Variants of haemophilia B. *Thromb. Diath. Haemorrh. 28*, 489 (1972).
19. Pfueller, S., J. B. Somer and P. A. Castaldi, Haemophilia B due to an abnormal factor IX. *Coagulation 2*, 213 (1969).
20. Osterud, B., *Personal communication* (1974).
21. Andreassen, M., Haemofili i Danmark. *Disputats*, Copenhagen (1943).
22. Révész, Th., Discordant identical twins. *The practitioner 210*, 162 (1973).
23. Frota-Pessoa, O., E. L. Gomes and Th. R. Calicchio, Christmas factor: Dosage compensation and the production of blood coagulation factor IX. *Science 139*, 348 (1962).
24. Lyon, M. L., Gene action in the X-chromosome of the mouse (Mus musculus L.). *Nature* (Lond.) *190*, 372 (1961).
25. Veltkamp, J. J., E. F. Drion and E. A. Loeliger, Detection of the carrier state in hereditary coagulation disorders. I. *Thromb. Diath. Haemorrh. 19*, 297 (1968).
Detection of the carrier state in hereditary coagulation disorders. II. *Thromb. Diath. Haemorrh. 19*, 404 (1968).
26. Gugler, E., S. Rosin and R. Bütler, Gerinnungsphysiologische Untersuchungen bei heterozygoten Anlageträgerinnen der Hämophilie. *Schweiz. med. Wschr. 10*, 320 (1965).
27. Nillson, I. M. and L. Holmberg, Haemophilia carriers. *Lancet 2*, 646 (1974).
28. Prentice, C. R. M. and C. D. Forbes, Hemophilia carriers. *Lancet 2*, 403 (1974).
29. Editorial. *Lancet 2*, 87 (1974).
30. Ekert, H., H. Helliger and P. H. Muntz, Detection of carriers of haemophilia. *Thromb. Diath. heamorrh. 30*, 255 (1973).
31. Denson, K. W. E., The detection of factor-VIII-like antigen in haemophilia carriers and in patients with raised levels of biologically active factor VIII. *Brit. J. Haemat. 24*, 451 (1973).
32. Meyer, D., G. M. Sitar, J. P. Allain, A. Plas and M. J. Larrieu, Problems in the detection of carriers of hemophilia A. In press (1975).

33. Bouma, B. N., M. M. van der Klaauw, J. J. Veltkamp, A. E. Starkenburg, N. H. van Tilburg and J. Hermans, Evaluation of the detection rate of hemophilia carriers. In press (1975).
34. Guttman, I., *Statistical tolerance region*. McGriffin, London (1970).

DISCUSSION

PAPER OF J.J. VELTKAMP C.S.

Anders: I would like to ask about the variability of the bleeder property and the constancy of different values in families.

Veltkamp: Yes, that is the same. The most recent study on this subject was done by D. F. Roberts and he found a very high degree of correlation between haemophiliac patients within the same family.

Anders: And what about the carrier examination in these families with a relatively high activity?

Veltkamp: In general, we only have experience with carriers of severe haemophilia; when you examine carriers with mild haemophilia, you find on average a somewhat higher activity.

Muller: Has the time come for screening mothers of haemophiliac patients to find out whether they are carriers?

Veltkamp: Yes, and if they want to have another child, you should send them to Galjaard.

Eriksson: How many of the patients are spontaneous mutations?

Veltkamp: We see spontaneous mutations in about 30% of our material for haemophilia A as well as haemophilia B. The mutation rate has been calculated, but this was done at a time that the genetic heterogeneity was not known and so the mutation rate figures were much too high. Probably, there are so many alleles which can give haemophilia that it does not make sense to do these calculations.

FAMILY DETECTION OF GENETIC DISEASES*

A. G. MOTULSKY

Health systems in most countries are constituted so that medical practitioners are responsible for diagnosis and treatment of illness in individual patients while public health departments are charged with health maintenance in the population-at-large. When a patient presents to a doctor, current practices will focus on the problems of that patient. Rarely, with certain infectious diseases of potential threat to the community, the physician will notify the public health department which may investigate contacts-at-risk.

Hereditary diseases present a new set of problems. For many diseases the mechanism of heredity is such that relatives are at high risk to be affected. Such relatives may 'carry' the disease in its early stages and not yet know about it; in others the 'carrier state' may cause little or no harm but place current and future children at high risk for the disease. The aim of family detection therefore is treatment of potentially life threatening genetic disease in affected relatives who do not know they are affected. In other cases, prevention of disease may be possible and, in some instances, genetic counseling and reproductive advice including intrauterine diagnosis and selective abortion can be provided to family members whose children are at risk. Search for diseases among relatives of patients affected with genetic disease has high yields when compared with programs aimed at disease in the community-at-large. Regardless of the rarity of the disease in the population, the family risks are very significant. Representative figures are listed in Table 1.

Table 2 lists a group of genetic diseases where identification of family members carrying this disease is mandatory. An additional group of genetic endocrine diseases is listed in Table 3. Specific prevention or treatment measures in affected family members can be practiced in all these diseases

* This contribution is an abstract of the lecture as it was given by Dr. Motulsky. This work was supported by NIH grant GM 15253.

Table 1. Risks for genetic diseases in families.

Mode of Inheritance	First degree relatives at risk	Risk	Other relatives at risk	Risk
Autosomal dominant	Sibs, children/parent (both sexes)	50%	Nephews and nieces Uncles, aunts, and cousins	25% 12.5%
Autosomal recessive	Sibs (both sexes)	25%	Nephews, nieces, uncles, aunts, and cousins	Usually less than 1%
X linked recessive	Brothers Sisters (carriers)	50%* 50%*	Maternal uncle Maternal aunt (carrier) Maternal male cousins Maternal female cousins (carriers)	50%* 50%* 25%* 25%*
Polygenic: Birth defects	Sibs, children	3-5%		<1%
Hypertension and diabetes	Sibs, children	5-15%		<5%

* Risks are negligible when the disease in an affected patient is caused by a new mutation. In general, with X-linked genetic lethal diseases such as Duchenne muscular dystrophy, one-third of all cases are due to new mutations.

with good results. These lists illustrate the falsity of the common misconception that genetic disease cannot be treated.

Table 4 refers to several conditions which can cause drug reactions because of genetic biochemical defects and require family testing to prevent those reactions in affected family members.

Table 5 documents several diseases where early detection in family members is possible but no specific treatment is available. However, early identification of affected patients allows such persons to make more meaningful reproductive decisions and allows better planning of their lives knowing that serious illness will develop in later life. Nevertheless, many families and their physicians may not choose to pursue family investigations in these disorders.

Table 6 lists a group of disorders where search for carriers should be done to identify relatives who will be quite well but whose genetic constitution places them at high risk to transmit a disease to their children. In some cases, intrauterine diagnosis with selective abortion may be possible. In others, only genetic counseling regarding the risks for the birth of affected children is feasible.

Table 2. Treatable or preventable inherited disorders for which search in family members of affected patients is mandatory.

Disorder	Mode of inheritance	Age of onset	Method of diagnosis	Treatment	Advantages of early diagnosis and treatment
Hemochromatosis	Autosomal dominant (autosomal recessive?)	Middle-aged adults	Liver biopsy most reliable	Venesection	Prevents liver, heart, and pancreatic disease
Bilateral retinoblastoma	Autosomal dominant	Infancy	Ophthalmoscopy	Eye enucleation	Prevents death
Hereditary spherocytosis	Autosomal dominant	Infancy to adult	Incubated osmotic fragility	Splenectomy	Prevents anemia and gallstones. Protects against splenic rupture
Hereditary polyposis	Autosomal dominant	Adulthood	Colonoscopy	Colectomy	Prevents colon cancer
Wilson's disease	Autosomal recessive	Childhood	Copper metabolism studies, liver biopsy most reliable	Remove copper by penicillamine	Prevents liver and brain damage
Familial hypercholesterolemia	Autosomal dominant	Infancy – coronary heart disease in adults	Cholesterol elevation (xanthomas frequent)	Diet, lipid lowering drugs	Prevents coronary heart disease*
Hypertension	Polygenic	Middle age	Blood pressure measurement	Antihypertensive drugs	Prevents heart, kidney, brain, eye disease
Diabetes	Polygenic	Throughout life	Urine glucose, glucose tolerance tests	Insulin, diet, (drugs)?	Prevents diabetic complications*

* Treatment not proven to be effective.

Table 3. Treatable or preventable inherited endocrine disorders for which search in family members of affected patients is mandatory*.

Disorder	Modes of inheritance	Age of onset	Method of diagnosis	Treatment	Advantages of early diagnosis and treatment
Diabetes insipidus, vasopressin-resistant type	X-linked recessive	Infancy	Urine concentration tests	Adequate hydration; chlorothiazide	Prevent mental retardation
Familial panhypopituitarism	Autosomal recessive; X-linked recessive	Infancy	Measurement of pituitary, adrenal, gonadal, and thyroid hormone	Replace deficient hormones	Prevent dwarfism, cretinism, adrenal insufficiency, gonadal failure
Isolated growth hormone deficiency	Autosomal recessive; autosomal dominant	Childhood	Measurement of growth hormone responses	Growth hormone	Prevent dwarfism
Pituitary hypogonadism	X-linked recessive; autosomal recessive	Adolescence	Plasma FSH, LH, testosterone	Testosterone	Prevent eunuchoidism
Primary male hypogonadism	X-linked recessive	Adolescence	Plasma FSH, LH, testosterone	Testosterone	Prevent eunuchoidism
Hypoparathyroidism	X-linked recessive; autosomal recessive	Infancy; adolescence	Serum calcium, phosphorus, parathyroid hormone	Calcium lactate; vitamin D	Prevent cataracts and tetany
Hyperparathyroidism	Autosomal dominant	Adulthood	Serum calcium, phosphorus, parathyroid hormone	Parathyroidectomy	Prevent renal damage and other complications of hypercalcemia
Vitamin-D-resistant rickets	X-linked dominant	Infancy	Serum calcium, phosphorus, alkaline phosphatase; measurement of urine TRP	Vitamin D (high doses); oral phosphate	Prevent rickets
Familial goiters	Autosomal recessive	Infancy; childhood	PBI; perchlorate test; measurement of iodotyrosines in urine; audiogram	Thyroxine	Prevent cretinism

Table 3. continued.

Disorder	Mode of inheritance	Age of onset	Method of diagnosis	Treatment	Advantages of early diagnosis and treatment
Hereditary form of athyrotic cretinism	Autosomal recessive	Infancy	PBI	Thyroxine	Prevent cretinism
Adrenogenital syndromes	Autosomal recessive	Infancy	Urinary 17-ketosteroids, pregnanetriol; buccal smear; serum electrolytes	Cortisone acetate	Prevent adrenal crises and avoid sex identification problems
Adrenal insufficiency	Autosomal recessive; autosomal dominant; X-linked recessive	Infancy; adolescence; adulthood	Serum cortisol, ACTH	Cortisone acetate, DOC	Prevent adrenal crises
Aldosterone deficiency	Autosomal recessive	Infancy; childhood	Serum electrolytes; measurement of aldosterone secretion	DOC	Prevent hyperkalemia and dehydration
Leucine-sensitive hypoglycemia	Autosomal recessive	Infancy	Blood sugar; measurements of plasma insulin responses	Low protein diet; diazoxide	Prevent convulsions
Multiple endocrine adenomatosis	Autosomal dominant	Adulthood	Serum calcium, phosphorus, blood sugar; gastrointestinal series	Parathyroidectomy; pancreatectomy; ulcer surgery	Prevent complications of hyperparathyroidism, hypoglycemia, peptic ulcer, metastatic cancer
Medullary thyroid carcinoma-pheochromocytoma syndromes	Autosomal dominant	Adulthood	Plasma calcitonin; measurement of blood pressure	Prophylactic thyroidectomy; removal of pheochromocytoma	Prevent thyroid carcinoma and complications of hypertension

* From Goldstein, J. L. and A. G. Motulsky, Genetics and endocrinology. In: *Textbook of endocrinology.* 5th ed., edited by R. H. Williams, Saunders Philadelphia 1974.

Table 4. Pharmacogenetic disorders for which search in family members of affected patients is advisable.

Disorder	Mode of inheritance	Drugs involved	Drug reaction	Method of diagnosis	Population at risk
Pseudocholines-terase deficiency	Autosomal recessive	Suxamethonium	Prolonged apnea	Pseudocholines-terase assay	Whites, very rare in Orientals and Blacks
G6PD deficiency	X linked	Many oxidant drugs	Hemolysis	G6PD assay	Originating from sub-tropical and tropical countries
'S. African' porphyria	Autosomal dominant	Barbiturates	Precipitates latent disease	Stools for porphyrins	S. Africans of Dutch origin

Table 6. Genetic diseases – carrier detection* advisable for reproductive decisions.

Disorder	Mode of inheritance	Age of onset	Method of carrier diagnosis	Preventive measures in carriers	Population affected
Duchenne muscular dystrophy	X-linked	Childhood	CPK level	Amniocentesis for male sex	All
Hemophilia	X-linked	Infancy to childhood	AHG level	Amniocentesis for male sex	All
Lesch-Nyhan syndrome	X-linked	Childhood	HGPRT assay	Amniocentesis – chromosomal study	All
Translocation (D/G) Down's syndrome	Empirical recurrence risks apply	Infancy	Chromosomal tests for balanced carrier	Amniocentesis – chromosomal study	All
Sickle cell anemia	Autosomal recessive	Infancy to childhood	Hemoglobin electrophoresis	Genetic counseling	Blacks
Thalassemia major	Autosomal recessive	Infancy to childhood	Red cell abnormalities, Hb A-2 increased	Genetic counseling	Mediterranean and tropical populations
Tay-Sachs disease	Autosomal recessive	Infancy	Hexosaminidase A assay	Amniocentesis – hexosaminidase assay	Ashkenazi Jews

* Limited to X-linked, recessive diseases, translocation Down's syndrome, and *frequent* autosomal recessive diseases. Detection of carriers for many rare inborn errors associated with enzyme deficiency is possible but the risk for normal sibs of affected patients to have affected offspring is very small since the frequency of the carrier state for such inborn errors is very low in the population.

Table 5. Disorders allowing early detection – no treatment or prevention possible.

Disorder	Mode of inheritance	Age of onset	Method of diagnosis
Polycystic kidneys	Autosomal dominant	Middle-aged adults	I.V.P. and other renal tests
Huntington's chorea	Autosomal dominant	Middle-aged adults	Careful neurological examination, history.
Cardiomyo-pathy	Autosomal dominant	Young adults	ECG, cardiology work up

Family detection of genetic disease ideally should be practiced by the physician or medical geneticist who identified the index patient. With large countries and widely spread families such as in the United States, there are many logistical problems in arranging for the appropriate tests. In smaller countries with a more centralized health system such as The Netherlands, there are fewer difficulties. It has been suggested to involve health departments in the activities of tracing family members-at-risk, particularly if it concerns a serious disease that can be treated or prevented.

Definite medical and legal rules in this field are lacking. Does failure to follow up relatives constitute malpractice? On the contrary, some persons might consider such identification as an invasion of privacy. Common sense needs to be used. It is a good idea to discuss the family situation with the index patient for advice regarding the advisability of family contacts. In most cases, no difficulties arise.

REFERENCES

McKusick's catalog Mendelian traits (McKusick, V. A., *Mendelian inheritance in man.* 4th ed., Johns Hopkins Press, Baltimore 1975) should be consulted for short descriptions and references to all diseases cited in this article.

DISCUSSION

PAPER OF A. G. MOTULSKY

Ten Kate: You have estimated the risk for relatives of, for example, cystic fibrosis patients to be less than 1%. We are always giving risk figures for one child, but most families have more than one child and I have just made a little calculation which indicates that if you are thinking of three children, the risk will be almost 2%.

Motulsky: Well, as you pointed out, a risk of 2% is still fortunately much lower than one of 15 to 25%, but it approaches the order of something you need to worry about. Unfortunately, as you discussed this morning, the tests we have for cystic fibrosis are not very good, and we really do not know at this point who is a carrier or not. Much work is going on in carrier detection of cystic fibrosis, so that I am personally confident that in the next five years we will have a test. Then, and certainly for the common diseases, one probably should test further to find the people at risk. It is particularly for cystic fibrosis, which in fact is rather common, probably the most common disease in European populations, for sickle cell anaemia in black populations, and for thalassaemia in the appropriate Mediterranean populations, and so on, that one probably should do more studies for the reasons that you mentioned.

Tan: What would you do if some life insurance company asked you about someone without his consent?

Motulsky: Well, I would never give anything to a life insurance company. If the company knew that I had seen the patient, the patient would have to give permission. If he does, I guess that as a physician I would have to supply this information, so in that sense perhaps the patient made a mistake in coming to me. We all know about this; it is one of the dilemmas we face with increasing knowledge of this sort, there are all kinds of information that we get to know about ourselves and our relatives, and which the rest of society might get to know, that in fact might hurt us in the long run. This is one of the real dilemmas of genetic medicine.

Galjaard: You said that when you find an abnormality and there is a possibility of relatives being affected or being a carrier, you would ask the patient first. Is that something you would insist on? I think of a translocation carrier whose sister is already pregnant.

Motulsky: Yes; actually, I do not recall any instances where patients have refused. Usually we spend quite some time with them and explain matters to them. I have heard from other people about situations where there were feuds within the family; they did not want to go and tell the rest of the family what had happened to the patient, and then you are in real difficulties. People have bypassed the patient and done it on the quiet, but I discussed some of these things with lawyers and it is a very murky area.

GENETIC COUNSELING: PRESENT STATUS
AND FUTURE PROSPECTS*

C. J. EPSTEIN

DEFINITIONS

Over the past few years I have had several occasions to write or to participate in conferences on genetic counseling. Faced with the task of writing once again on the subject, it is of interest to look back at the definitions of genetic counseling which were used earlier. In a talk given in 1972, I stated that:

'Genetic counseling is the science – and the art – of preventing genetic disease. So defined, the term included not only the more conventional types of counseling. . . but all procedures which lead to the elimination of genetic disorders.' (Epstein, 1974).

A similar concept was set forth, more succinctly, in the introduction to a text-book chapter on medical genetics written shortly thereafter.

'The principal purpose of genetic counseling is the prevention of genetically determined disorders. This is usually accomplished by the provision of information concerning risks of occurrence or recurrence.' (Epstein, 1975).

And, on yet another occasion I wrote:

'Genetic counseling is the process of providing information about the risk of occurrence and recurrence of genetic disease and, when appropriate, of taking steps to modify these risks. . . Counseling has both a passive component – the giving of risks – and an active one – the modification of these risks.' (Epstein, 1973).

In all of these definitions there is a two-fold emphasis, one on the provision of information – usually in the form of risk figures, and the second on the

* Supported in part by grants from the National Foundation – March of Dimes, The National Institute of General Medical Sciences (GM-19,527), and the Maternal and Child Health Service (Project No. 445).

prevention of genetic disorders. Although the text accompanying all of these definitions included a discussion of the psychological aspects of genetic disease and of the counseling process, it is clear, in retrospect, that the two objectives just mentioned were the major ones.

Contrast, now, the three definitions set forth above with two others. The first is from a WHO report on the prevention, treatment, and rehabilitation of genetic disorders:

'The role of the genetic counselor should be to assist the physician with diagnosis, to estimate the recurrence risk, to interpret this information to the patient in meaningful terms, and to help the patient to reach and act upon an appropriate decision.' (WHO Scientific Group, 1972)

A new element is introduced by this definition, that of helping the patient decide what to do with the information that is provided. This element is greatly amplified in the next and last definition, one devised by a large committee of American and Canadian physicians and scientists:

'Genetic counseling is a communication process which deals with the human problems associated with the occurrence, or the risk of occurrence, of a genetic disorder in a family. This process involves an attempt by one or more appropriately trained persons to help the individual or family (1) comprehend the medical facts, including the diagnosis, the probable course of the disorder, and the available management; (2) appreciate the way heredity contributes to the disorder, and the risk of recurrence in specified relatives; (3) understand the options for dealing with the risk of recurrence; (4) choose the course of action which seems appropriate to them in view of their risk and the family goals and act in accordance with that decision; and (5) make the best possible adjustment to the disorder in an affected family member and/or to the risk of recurrence of that disorder.' (Fraser, 1974)

In this definition there is no mention of the *prevention* of genetic disease. The emphasis is now on *counseling* – 'a communication process. . . to help the individual or family comprehend. . . appreciate. . . understand. . . choose. . . act. . . make the best possible adjustment.'

Since I was a member of the committee which drew up this definition, one quite different from the first three of my own devising, I now find myself trying to decide just what I really think genetic counseling is. Otherwise, how can I discuss its present status and future prospects?

SHIFTS IN EMPHASIS

In a sense, all definitions are self serving, since they are usually intended to support the biases, practices, and areas of interest and expertise of those who devise them – and I certainly do not exclude myself. Thus, the increasing emphasis on counseling represents the entrance into the field of genetic counseling, as it is currently being practiced, of increasing numbers of persons with backgrounds in counseling *per se* rather than in the strictly medical and genetic aspects of genetic disease. But, this is certainly not the whole or necessarily even the principal explanation. It is clear in my own case and, I suspect, the cases of many of the medically trained genetic counselors, that the prevention of genetic disease has ceased to be the overriding objective or the proper measure of genetic counseling, and there are several reasons for this.

ATTAINABILITY OF PREVENTION AS A GOAL

First, there is the realization that, certainly in the reasonably foreseeable future and probably in the long range future as well, prevention of all or even most genetically determined defects is an unattainable goal. This unattainability is either a theoretical one resulting from the lack of any means of actually preventing the disorder or a practical one resulting from an inability to make existing means of prevention available or from a resistance on the part of the persons at risk to their use. These concepts can be illustrated by reference to figure 1. The assumptions on which this figure is based are discussed in greater detail in an earlier paper (Epstein, 1974) but will be briefly summarized here. Except for Down's syndrome, in which women over 40 are advised not to have children, counseling of the 'past' refers purely to the retrospective type of risk-giving counseling. This is the counseling given after an affected child has been born. Its impact on the total incidence of diseases or conditions with chromosomal, single gene, and polygenic (or, better, multifactorial) etiologies is minimal. By contrast, genetic counseling of the 'present', which includes the use of amniocentesis and selective abortion for chromosomal and suspected biochemical disorders and of anti-Rh-immune globulin to prevent sensitization to the Rh factor, is capable of reducing the total incidence of genetic disorders by 20 to 25%. The major residuals are in the various presently undetectable polygenic or multifactorial disorders, the single gene disorders for which no heterozygote

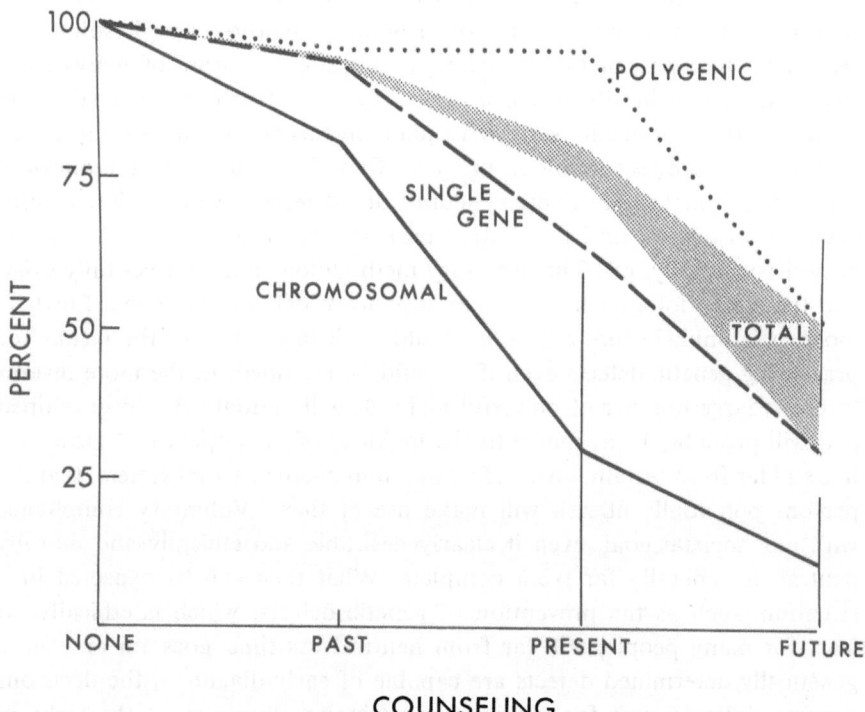

Fig. 1. The effect of genetic counseling on the incidence of genetically determined birth defects. Reprinted from Epstein, 1974.

or *in utero* diagnostic procedures are available or which arise as new muta-tions, and the chromosomal disorders, such as XXX and XYY, for which abortion might not be considered as indicated. It is, of course, of interest to note that the 'present' of two years ago, when this figure was prepared, is not the 'present' of now. For example, reasonably good means for the intrauterine diagnosis of neural tube defects, which did not exist then, are now available (Brock and Sutcliffe, 1972).

The projections for the future were based on prenatal monitoring of all pregnancies by chromosome analysis, fetal visualization, and improved biochemical methods, and on the possible role of environmental manipula-tion in the prevention of multifactorial disorders. Using the most reasonable assumptions I could, I estimated that there would still be a residual non-preventable incidence of 30 to 50% of genetically determined disorders. This is clearly a tenuous estimate, since it is very much influenced by what is included in the definition of genetically determined disease and what preventive means one is capable of visualizing. Nevertheless, it still seems reasonable to expect that even with very sophisticated means of analysis and treatment, there will still be defects or disorders which will not be preventable.

Even if these projections are reasonable in theory, the question arises of whether they are reasonable in practice. Can all pregnancies be monitored for chromosomal abnormalities, neural tube defects, a wide variety of bio-chemical disorders, and gross structural defects? For the near future the answer is certainly, no! The necessary methodology does not yet fully exist, and the methodology which does exist is not widely disseminated. Further-more, it is unlikely that everyone would avail themselves of the means for preventing genetic defects even if it could be provided. In the more distant future, a large number of powerful methods will undoubtedly be developed and will probably be available to the majority of the population. However, it is still far from certain, given a free and non-coercive social system, that the persons potentially at risk will make use of them. Voluntary compliance with any societal goal, even if clearly desirable and ethically and morally neutral, is generally far from complete. What then can be expected in a situation, such as the prevention of genetic defects, which is ethically, at least for many people, still far from neutral? As time goes on and more genetically determined defects are capable of early diagnosis, the decisions become difficult even for the more doctrinaire advocates of the right of parents to have perfectly normal or healthy children. It is easy to lump together all genetically determined or influenced abnormalities and diseases under the rubric 'genetic abnormality' and to advocate their prevention as long as one is not able to do anything about them. However, once the means for prevention become available, it becomes necessary to decide what situations ought to be prevented and which, if any, ought not. At present there is still considerable indecision about what ought be done with XXX and XXY fetuses and with fetuses diagnosed as having galactosemia – a supposedly treatable disease. What dilemmas will exist, then, when it becomes possible to diagnose *in utero* a cleft lip and palate or coarctation of the aorta or polydactyly or diabetes mellitus or hypercholesterolemia?

OTHER REASONS FOR SHIFT TOWARDS COMMUNICATION

Since I do not feel that it is fruitful, in the present discussion, to pursue this line of inquiry further, I shall briefly summarize it and then return to a further consideration of the reasons for a shift in emphasis from prevention to communication in the definition of genetic counseling. At present, total prevention of genetic abnormalities is a practical and theoretical impossibility; in the future, the theoretical limitations will become less, although they will not disappear, and the practical problems will continue to persist. One of these practical problems will be an ethical one, and this brings us to the second reason for the diminishing primacy of genetic disease prevention in genetic counseling: not all individuals at risk of transmitting a genetic disorder, particularly a relatively mild one, are anxious to prevent its occurrence. While the prevention of genetic disease or defects might in many instances appear to be desirable to the counselor, it is by no means certain that the persons at risk will always be of the same opinion – the means of prevention may not be acceptable, or the family may only want information, not action. In situations such as this, it is generally felt that it is incumbent upon the counselor not to interpose his own personal opinions into the counseling situation. This feeling has been given expression in the notion that counseling should be non-directive. As a practical matter it is rarely possible for the counseling to be wholly non-directive, even if the counselor tried to make it so. Biases are generally communicated, if only unconsciously. In addition, the patient frequently asks for a direct statement of the counselor's opinion of what ought to be done and will not accept a purely objective recitation of facts and figures. My own feeling is that totally non-directive counseling is unattainable and, for most patients, is not really desirable. However, there is a point beyond which the counselor should not go, and that is the point at which he becomes the advocate of a position which the patient is unable, for whatever reasons, to accept. In actuality, none of this should become a problem and the question of directive versus non-directive counseling becomes moot if the counseling is sufficiently thorough to permit the patients or parents to make the choice of a course of action stipulated in the fifth definition.

Conversely, even if a family or patient is willing to accept prevention of a genetically determined defect as his primary reason for obtaining genetic counseling, the need for sufficient and appropriate counseling cannot be underestimated. This has been forcefully emphasized to me by the results of inquiries made to women (as well as to their husbands) who have undergone therapeutic abortion after the prenatal diagnosis of chromosomal or metabolic abnormalities or of the male sex when the woman was a carrier of an X-linked disease (Blumberg and Golbus 1974). There is no question that this group was as greatly interested as anyone, including the counselors themselves, in seeking to prevent the birth of a genetically abnormal child. However, unlike the counselor who advocates or at least supports the concept without being personally involved, it is the woman at risk who has to undergo the physical trauma of an abortion and both she and her husband who are confronted with the psychological trauma. In retrospect, it was certainly naive for us to have expected the latter to be anything but profound, but it certainly was. Severe post-abortion depressions were the rule, and serious tension between the marital partners, sometimes leading to temporary separations, was not infrequent. Neither we nor the family was prepared for what was to occur, and, unfortunately, we were not there to help them when it did. I do not wish to suggest that selective abortion for genetic reasons necessarily produces irreversible psychological damage. Several women who underwent such abortions deliberately became pregnant and went through the prenatal diagnostic procedure again. Nevertheless, it is clear that the amount of counseling required, at all stages of the process, is considerably greater than any of us would have anticipated, and that prevention of disease is not enough.

Last in our list of reasons why emphasis on prevention *per se* has diminished is the realization that very often the problem is not what to do in the future but what should be done about something that has already occurred. Here we are discussing genetic counseling in its most restricted sense, that type of counseling which is essentially retrospective and initiated after the birth of an abnormal child. While the parental concerns are frequently expressed in terms of risks of occurrence and recurrence, the unstated and frequently much deeper concerns center around the affected child itself and the ways in which they, the parents, may have produced or contributed to its problem. Although genetic counselors have, in general, been cognizant of these problems, they have not been aware of what is actually required to deal with them in a constructive manner. A single visit to a genetic clinic is rarely enough, even if the diagnosis is straightforward and the risks easy to calculate and state. In some cases, two visits may suffice, often three or more are necessary. No matter how many visits, in what form, or with whom, it is no longer sufficient merely to acknowledge the concept of handling the psychological consequences of genetic abnormalities. These consequences must, in fact, be handled.

AIMS OF GENETIC COUNSELING

There is no question that the increased emphasis on counseling is a healthy and long overdue development. However, this shift in emphasis has had some curious consequences. For example, I was myself very recently told that because I do not possess the appropriate training and credentials in counseling, I am not a genetic counselor at all. A medical geneticist – yes; a counselor – no! There is a great irony in this, since two years ago I gave a talk in which I expressed exactly the contrary point of view: I, a physician trained in medical genetics, was *the* genetic counselor; all others, including those individuals whose training was in counseling and genetics, but not in medicine, were not! (Epstein 1973) Both of these statements were made in the context of who should be doing what in an overall genetic counseling situation and reflect, I am afraid, the difficulties that attempts to make semantic distinctions can get us into. The critical point is that our understanding of what genetic counseling is has changed markedly in the last few years, and it is important to recognize just what the concept really means. In a formal sense, the term 'genetic counseling' means just what it says – counseling with regard to genetic matters. Understood in this way, the last of the definitions set forth above – 'genetic counseling is a communication process. . .' is an excellent definition of what is included. However, I feel, even though I was associated with its genesis, that this definition is too restrictive in its connotations. With its major emphasis on communication, it appears to separate counseling *per se* from the other aspects of what might be called the diagnosis, management and prevention of genetic disorders, and I do not believe this separation is either warranted or useful. But, rather than attempt another formal definition of a term which may already have outlived its usefulness, even though I have no better one to suggest in its place, I shall try to identify what I believe to be the present aims of genetic counseling as understood in a broader and less restrictive sense.

PRESENTATION OF INFORMATION: PASSIVE COUNSELING

The aims of genetic counseling can be divided into three components. Although each does not necessarily apply in every instance, all three do fit within the overall concept. The first component is the obtaining and presentation of the relevant medical and genetic information. Included in this are the proper diagnosis of genetic disorders and traits, the estimation of genetic risks of occurrence and recurrence, and the transmission of these diagnoses and estimates to the concerned individuals. The elements of diagnosis, risk calculation, and information transfer are all included in this aim and are integral aspects of the counseling situation. Counseling does not begin after the diagnosis is made – the making of the diagnosis, with the taking of the medical history and the necessary physical and laboratory examinations, are essential ·parts of the counseling process. The same is true of the taking of the family history or pedigree and of the calculation of genetic risks when these are required. Furthermore, since appropriate counseling requires accurate facts, it is implicit in this formulation that it is the obligation of the counselor or counselors to certify the accuracy of these facts. The counselor must take direct responsibility for the accuracy of his information, whether he obtains it himself or from others. Otherwise, because of the rarity of many of the conditions dealt with and the complexity of many of the laboratory tests which may be required, there is a very real danger that erroneous information will be transmitted.

ACTIVE COUNSELING

As I have described it, the first component of genetic counseling is essentially a *passive* one – one which is generally initiated after the appearance or recognition, whether at birth or later, of an individual who has some problem which may be genetic in origin and terminates with the presentation of information. By contrast, the second component of genetic counseling is an *active* one in which there is some form of direct intervention to *reduce* the risk of occurrence of genetically determined abnormalities. It is this notion of active counseling that is contained, perhaps in too bald a fashion, within the earlier definitions of genetic counseling and which is not, unfortunately, really part of the latter ones. Again, the concept is that these active means of risk reduction are part of genetic counseling rather than being separate from it. This is not only because genetic problems are being dealt with, but also because the same constraints of accuracy and responsibility as apply to the first, passive component apply here as well – and because the third component of genetic counseling, the psychological one, is also inextricably involved.

SCREENING

Included in the second, active component of genetic counseling are such procedures as population screening and prenatal diagnosis with selective abortion. The screening of populations for genetic purposes falls into several categories, of which the principal ones are screening for medical management, screening for reproductive advice, and screening for purposes of enumeration (Committee on Screening for Inborn Errors of Metabolism, 1975). The first of these is best exemplified by the many programs for detection of phenylketonuria and often other metabolic diseases in the neonatal period. However, similar programs are contemplated for conditions, such as hypercholesterolemia, which do not have deleterious effects until later in life. While the main objective of this type of screening program is to permit early therapy prior to the occurrence of irreversible damage, the fact that genetic conditions are involved immediately necessitates appropriate counseling of the 'passive' type with regard to recurrence risks, etiology, and potential effects in other family members.

PRENATAL DIAGNOSIS

Screening for reproductive advice is the most direct extension of conventional genetic counseling. In the United States this type of screening program has been applied mainly to the detection of carriers of sickle cell anemia in the Black population and of Tay-Sachs disease in the Ashkenazi Jewish group. At the moment, the latter is perhaps the most effective screening program since the population at risk is well defined, the tests (for serum hexosaminidase activity) are reliable, and relatively inexpensive and effective means for acting on the information are available (Kaback and Zeiger 1972). These means are, of course, the prenatal determination of the enzymological status of the fetus and, if the fetus is affected and the parents so desire, selective therapeutic abortion. Prenatal diagnosis has been mentioned several times in this discussion, and I do not think further explication is required. However, the one point that I would make here is that the prenatal diagnosis of genetic disorders is very much a form of genetic counseling. While it employs obstetrical techniques for obtaining the samples required for analysis and, if necessary, for termination of the pregnancy, the purposes of the procedure are genetic and the same considerations as apply to other forms of genetic counseling are still relevant. It is likely that in the future other techniques, such as artificial insemination, which is already in limited use for genetic purposes, and *in vitro* fertilization and/or ovum transfer will also be numbered among the methods of active genetic counseling.

PSYCHOLOGICAL ASPECTS OF COUNSELING

The third component of genetic counseling – counseling in the psychological sense – has already been discussed in some detail. As has been pointed out, while it does not in itself represent anything that can be considered as a new innovation, the recognition accorded to it is distinctly new. In our own genetic counseling unit we find that increasing time is being spent in this activity. It is rapidly becoming routine for all of our patients to be seen prior to the actual medical session or sessions by one of the non-physician members of the genetics group. While part of this visit is devoted to the obtaining of a family history and other pertinent information, the time is also spent in other activities which we believe are of great value. These include an assessment of the family or patient's expectations and real desires with regard to the genetic counseling, an allaying of fears and the correction of misconceptions about the medical aspects of the counseling process, and the establishment of a relationship which can be carried on beyond the purely medical and genetic aspects of the process. The physician-medical geneticist, when he becomes the deliverer of 'bad news' – either in the form of a diagnosis or of genetic risks – can often no longer relate effectively with the recipients of the information. The deliverer becomes identified with the information he delivers. The person who sees the patient or family prior to the receipt of such information is in an excellent position then to work with him or them afterwards to assist in all of the many aspects in counseling outlined in the fifth definition: comprehension of facts, understanding of options, choice of a course of action, and adjustment to the situation. This assistance may require one visit, or it may require several.

In a sense this third component of counseling has many features which bring it close to psychotherapy, and I would not dispute that this is the case. However, the facts, the options, and the courses of action are medical and genetic, and for this reason I do not believe that the psychological component of genetic counseling, as long as it is devoted to assistance in decision making and adjustment to the specific genetic and medical situation, can be divorced from the other aspects that have been discussed. To the contrary, I feel that such psychological counseling can best be given within the framework of an integrated genetic counseling program.

Although the brief description of the role of the psychological component of counseling has been couched principally in terms of its relevance to the first 'passive' genetic component of genetic counseling, its role in the active forms of counseling, while perhaps somewhat different in form, cannot be lost sight of. The need for better psychological management with regard to prenatal diagnosis and abortion has already been mentioned. The same has also been found to be the case even in population screening programs aimed at heterozygote detection. What might seem to the geneticist to be a relatively straightforward piece of information – namely, that a person is the carrier of a gene for hemoglobin S or for hexosaminidase A deficiency – can have tremendous and often unappreciated psychological implications for the person so identified, and these implications must be properly dealt with.

In my description of how the psychological component of genetic counseling can or should be handled, I made frequent use of terms such as 'believe' and 'feel'. What I have said constitutes a summary of my own beliefs and feelings, ones which are shared with others but which have certainly not been validated in any objective sense. And, even if it is granted that psychological counseling is a valid component of genetic counseling, it is by no means clear how it should best be done or how its effectiveness can be assessed. Useful measures of success in this area, as opposed to those for achieving a more concrete goal such as dissuading a couple from having children when the risk is high (Carter et al. 1971), have yet to be devised. This is not a problem unique to genetic counseling and applies to other situations in which evaluation of a psychotherapeutic process is desired. However, the relatively defined nature of genetic counseling should make it an excellent subject for careful analysis, and beginning steps in this direction are now being made in several quarters.

ORGANIZATION OF GENETIC COUNSELING

How can one best describe the present status of genetic counseling, assuming that it has the three components and the various characteristics that I have outlined above? Perhaps the most accurate statement that can be made is that genetic counseling is in a state of flux. The definitions and goals are changing rapidly, the techniques which can be employed are increasing in number, complexity, and power, and the general organization of genetic counseling is changing in form. The first two of these – definitions and goals, and techniques – have already been discussed at length – and I shall now turn my attention to the third, the organization of genetic counseling.

At the present time, the organization of genetic counseling services, at least in the United States, is relatively unsystematic, and large segments of the population do not have ready access to them. Genetic counseling of the more conventional type is performed by numerous individuals and groups located principally in major medical centers. Some of the groups act as comprehensive counseling organizations which deal with a wide range of problems and have all of the essential laboratory facilities at their disposal. Other groups and individuals are concerned with a more restricted range of problems, and several such groups or persons may coexist in the same institution without effective intercommunication. Often superimposed on these are screening programs, particularly for phenylketonuria and sickle cell trait, which may (although it is not necessary that they should) be totally removed from contact with experienced geneticists.

Just as there is no uniformity or systematization of how the services are provided, there is no uniformity or standards of training or performance for those who provide them. Individuals with a wide variety of professional training and experience are involved. Some are trained medical geneticists, while others are physicians without genetic training, basic geneticists, nurses, social workers, and genetic associates or assistants – the last a new group of individuals receiving special training in genetics and counseling techniques. Some are competent to provide good counseling, others are not.

PHILOSOPHY OF ORGANIZATION

However, despite his present state of relative disorganization, a general philosophy toward the organization of genetic counseling seems to be evolving. Implicit in this philosophy are two assumptions: the first is that genetic counseling in its broader aspects can no longer be handled by single persons operating in isolation. I have already spoken of the different roles played by those concerned primarily with medical and genetic matters and those involved with the more psychological aspects. The same also applies to the medical and genetic aspects *per se*, since it is no longer possible for a single individual to encompass, for example, cytogenetics, biochemical genetics, and identification of complex malformation syndromes, let alone also participate in screening programs and amniocentesis. The second assumption is that a correct diagnosis and assessment of genetic factors is fundamental to effective counseling. Since diagnosis still remains a medical task and the genetic assessment both relies on and may influence it, individuals trained in both medicine and genetics – medical geneticists – must participate in the counseling process. This does not mean that the counseling of many problems can not or should not be handled by persons lacking some of these qualifications. It does, however, mean that such persons are required in units handling the more complicated types of counseling problems.

CENTERS AND SATELLITES

The outcome of these two assumptions is that medical genetics is emerging as a specialty of medicine while, at the same time, genetic counseling units containing both medical geneticists and other types of appropriately trained personnel are being established. In virtually all cases, such units are being formed within large medical centers, affiliated to medical schools which can provide the many specialized diagnostic and consultative resources that are required. However, this type of localization of counseling units can lead to difficulties in making the counseling readily available to those who need it. While ready access to university medical centers may be possible in relatively small countries or geographical areas, this is clearly not the case in larger countries, such as the United States, in which medical schools may be located many hundreds of miles away from substantial residential areas. Two possible approaches to this problem can be envisioned. One is to have more of the counseling, at least for the simpler matters, handled by local physicians. For this to succeed, appropriate training of these individuals in the content and techniques of counseling is required, and our medical curricula and training programs are not yet oriented in this way. The other approach is for the centralized university-based groups to directly involve themselves in genetic counseling activities in more distant areas. This is a pattern which is gradually evolving in many areas of the United States and one with which we in San Francisco have been developing considerable experience (Epstein et al. 1975). The essence of our approach is to establish what we refer to as a center-satellite system: a large, comprehensive, university-based genetic counseling unit with a large number of affiliated community 'satellite' clinics. Some of these satellites, all of which are staffed by medical geneticists from the central clinic, are quite distant from the center but still benefit directly from the specialized laboratory resources and general expertise that is available there. It is presently our belief, and again I point out the lack of formal substantiation, that this type of system is capable of fulfilling four essential requirements for the delivery of genetic counseling services: *quality*, *availability*, *efficiency*, and *economic feasibility*.

FUTURE PROSPECTS

If all that I have discussed constitutes a fair summary of the present status of genetic counseling, what can be said of its future prospects? No matter what projections I might make based on present knowledge, it is possible, perhaps even likely that wholly unanticipated events will occur which will render many of these projections meaningless. In this regard it should be recalled that the technique of prenatal diagnosis, which did not enter the mainstream of genetic counseling until about 1967, has already resulted in great changes in our entire approach. Nevertheless, it is still possible to make some reasonable predictions about what is likely to happen in genetic counseling in the not too distant future. The predictions can be divided into two groups – those concerning organization and those relating to the technical aspects of counseling.

FUTURE ORGANIZATION

On the organizational side, I expect that medical genetics will emerge as a separate and recognized specialty of medicine, one which will have an identify of its own and separate from that of the other medical subspecialties. At the same time, it is likely that there will be increased interest and activity in the training of non-medical personnel (now referred to as genetic associates or assistants) to carry out many of the information gathering, information transmitting, and, in particular, psychological aspects of genetic counseling. These two types of people – medical geneticists and genetic associates (or their equivalents) – as well as others with specialized knowledge and skills – will be organized into comprehensive genetic counseling centers which will form the basis for the distribution of all components of genetic counseling. As a result, both genetic counseling itself and the various laboratory procedures and other specialized techniques (including population screening and prenatal diagnosis) which are part of it will be handled on a regionalized basis.

TECHNICAL POSSIBILITIES

While these organizational prospects flow quite directly from the earlier discussions, many of the predictions on the technical side do not, and require a somewhat more detailed discussion. There are, however, two developments in the technical aspects of genetic counseling which can be inferred from what has already been said. One is the introduction of better techniques for the psychological aspects of genetic counseling, and the other is the creation and use of appropriate measures for evaluating the effectiveness of genetic counseling in attaining its several goals. These two are interconnected, since the former, the introduction of better techniques, cannot really take place without the existence of valid mechanisms for evaluating the effectiveness of these techniques. Methods for interviewing and for the handling of emotional problems and crises already do exist, and it is their adaptation to and utilization in genetic counseling that is required. Likewise, relatively crude measurements of counseling effectiveness have already been applied and have yielded useful information (Leonard et al. 1972), but more incisive and sophisticated assessments which deal with the totality of the goals of counseling still await formulation and implementation.

AUTOMATION AND COMPUTERS

The greater utilization of automated techniques for biochemical analysis and cytogenetic analysis represent a technical change that has already begun. Urine and plasma amino acid analysis has long been performed by automated equipment, and the screening programs for heterozygosity for Tay-Sachs disease rely on automated instrumentation for enzyme assay and data processing (Delvin et al. 1974). Other types of automated biochemical analysis are now being developed, including high pressure liquid and gas-liquid chromatography. Success is already being achieved in the coupling of such chromatographic methods with mass spectrometry to allow the screening for and identification of unknown components in body fluids which may be etiologically relevant in genetic disorders (Jellum et al. 1971). The principal application of these techniques at present is in the identification of organic acids, but numerous other applications can be readily visualized.

Automation of cytogenetic procedures is less advanced but still holds considerable promise for the future. Progress is being made in several areas

– the location of metaphases on the slide, the enumeration of the metaphase chromosomes, the identification of the individual chromosomes and assessment of their normality. The last of these makes use of the finer analysis of the individual chromosomes now made possible by the various types of staining techniques and will, undoubtedly, be capable of much greater refinement and sensitivity than now exists. Furthermore, it is not unlikely that the techniques of cell culture required for preparation of chromosomes for analysis, perhaps the most tedious aspect of the entire procedure, will themselves be automated. This will become critical if much larger scale use of prenatal diagnosis occurs.

None of the automation just discussed would be possible without the use of computers for instrument operation and for data storage and retrieval. Other ways of using computers in genetic counseling are also being explored and are likely to become important in the future: the storage of records and pedigrees for individual patients and families, the creation of regional inter-linked genetic registries, and the facilitation of diagnosis by the storage and retrieval of information concerning complex developmental syndromes, chromosomal abnormalities, and the like. These capabilities will become essential as the number of identified genetic entities increases and as genetic counseling becomes available to larger segments of the population.

OTHER TECHNIQUES

There are still other technical advances that can be anticipated although the precise methodology to be used must still be developed. Included among these are improved methods for identification of heterozygosity for X-linked disorders, for metabolic diseases, and for incompletely penetrant autosomal dominantly inherited disorders. Such methods would also facilitate wider scale screening for persons at risk of having genetically abnormal offspring. In addition, there will undoubtedly be the identification of new and specific genetic entities within broad disease categories such as mental retardation, and the development of appropriate diagnostic criteria for them. Better empiric risk figures will be developed for conditions which are still not amenable to specific etiologic diagnoses. And, finally, new techniques for the prenatal diagnosis of genetic defects and other congenital abnormalities will be introduced. As has already been mentioned, it is likely that it will eventually be possible to learn a great deal about the fetus *in utero* and to diagnose developmental and other abnormalities which are not presently susceptible to analysis. This will come about by improvement of existing procedures, by the use of physical techniques of fetal visualization – either directly by optical means or indirectly by ultrasound and other noninvasive techniques, and by the development of molecular mechanisms for inducing the expression of genetic functions that are not ordinarily expressed.

TREATMENT

Except for brief reference to the screening for phenylketonuria for the purpose of initiating early treatment, nothing has been said about therapy *per se* as a component of genetic counseling. Given the rather broad view of genetic counseling that is being advanced here, particularly with regard to active aspects, it is difficult to draw a sharp line that distinguishes counseling from treatment. This difficulty is likely to increase in the future when more powerful techniques for preventing the development of the deleterious effects of genetic disorders are introduced. Nevertheless, for the moment, I feel that treatment itself is part of the general practice of medicine and is properly separated at least conceptually from genetic counseling as discussed here.

CONCLUSION

In concluding I would like to reiterate three points that I have already made. First, the total prevention of genetic diseases is an unattainable and perhaps even an unjustified goal of genetic counseling, and there has been a shift in emphasis from prevention to communication. Second, as a result of this, as well as of technical advances, genetic counseling is now in a state of flux – changing rapidly but hopefully evolving toward better forms and practices. And, finally, no matter what projections for the future we might make, it is likely that unanticipated occurrences will turn us in directions which cannot now be 'predicted' but which will continue to make genetic counseling an exciting and useful area of endeavour.

REFERENCES

1. Blumberg, B. and M. Golbus, Psychological sequelae of abortion performed for a genetic indication. *Amer. J. Hum. Genet. 26*, 15A (1974).
2. Brock, D. J. H. and R. G. Sutcliffe, Alpha-fetoprotein in the antenatal diagnosis of anencephaly and spina bifida. *Lancet 2*, 197-199 (1972).
3. Carter, C. O., K. A. Evans, J. A. Fraser Roberts and A. R. Buch, Genetic clinic: a follow up. *Lancet 1*, 281-285 (1971).
4. Committee on Screening for Inborn Errors of Metabolism. *Report to National Research Council*. National Academy of Science. In preparation (1975).
5. Delvin, E., A. Pottier, C. R. Scriver and R. J. M. Gold, The application of an automated hexosaminidase assay to genetic screening. *Clin. Chim. Acta 53*, 135-142 (1974).
6. Epstein, C. J., Who should do genetic counseling, and under what circumstances. In: *Contemporary Genetic Counseling*. Birth Defects Original Article Series 9: (4), 39-48 (1973).
7. Epstein, C. J., Genetic counseling – past, present and future, In: K. S. Moghissi (ed.), *Birth defects and fetal development, endocrine and metabolic factors* (C. C. Thomas, Springfield, Ill.) pp. 268-299 (1974).
8. Epstein, C. J., Genetic counseling. In: *The science and practice of clinical medicine*. (Grune and Stratton, New York) (1975).
9. Epstein, C. J., R. P. Erickson, B. D. Hall and M. S. Golbus, The center-satellite system for the wide-scale distribution of genetic counseling services. *Amer. J. Hum. Genet. 27*, 322-332 (1975).
10. Fraser, F. C., Genetic counseling. *Amer. J. Hum. Genet. 26*: 636-659 (1974).
11. Jellum, E., O. Stokke and L. Eldjarn, Screening for metabolic disorders using gas-liquid chromatography, mass spectrometry, and computer technique. *Scand. J. Clin. Lab. Invest. 27*, 273-285 (1971).
12. Kaback, M. M. and R. S. Zeiger, Heterozygote detection in Tay-Sachs disease: a prototype community screening program for the prevention of recessive genetic disorders. In: B. W. Volk and S. M. Aronson (eds.), *Sphingolipids, sphingolipidoses, and allied disorders*. (Plenum Press, New York), pp. 613-632 (1972).
13. Leonard, C. O., G. A. Chase and B. Childs, Genetic counseling: a consumer's view. *New Eng. J. Med. 287*, 433-439 (1972).
14. WHO Scientific Group, *Genetic disorders: prevention, treatment and rehabilitation*. World Health Organization Technical Report Series, No. 497, pp. 1-46 (1972).

DISCUSSION

PAPER OF C.J. EPSTEIN

Went: Since we have heard a view from over the ocean, we might also perhaps hear at least a comment from over the Channel?

Edwards: It is difficult to compare the American and the British system, because we have a more or less organized health service, with various defects, in Great Britain, and consequently we have the opportunity to integrate genetic counseling with the health service rather than setting up another system. Basically, if you do not have an organized medical service and you set up a system which *is* organized, it seems to me an extremely dangerous system. Because it will take over from whatever medical establishment there is, and I feel that in the long run one must try to integrate genetic counseling within medicine. It seems to me the most difficult field of medicine. There are large numbers of fields which are very simple and are being done by medically qualified people with a great inefficiency and loss of manpower. Examples of such fields include examination of normal children, baby clinics, contraception, and so on. While these things are being done by medically qualified people who are highly trained, all this seems to me to be very questionable. If I understand you correctly, you are suggesting that in this most difficult field you should use ancillary workers. In Britain I think we are trying to put this complicated field into the hands of those who are basically pediatricians and to solve the manpower problems by pushing semi-skilled work such as baby clinics, vaccination, contraception, and so on, into the hands of paramedical personnel. We are in a very fortunate position by having an integrated health service and to that extent we cannot comment on the American system. But there is a very big difference in genetic counseling, because it is all right if you stick to very rare diseases for which there is a specific genetic problem, but once you accept multifactorial disease you are in fact taking on the whole of disease; this seems to me to be a very big undertaking, to separate it from the conventional medical system. So I feel I am strategically departing from a completely different attitude. I would wish to integrate the genetic counseling within medicine, and if people say, well, doctors are too busy, or they are too expensive, or there are not enough of them well, then stop doing things which are not necessary, like examining healthy people, healthy children, and so on. So if you ask for a cross-channel view, this seems to me to be the central dichotomy. The example I wish to put forward, as an example of how things should be done and have been done, is the rhesus system. The rhesus disease was a purely genetical disease, its whole mechanism is genetical. It was discovered by the blood groupists, it was taken over by the obstetricians, it was handled really very efficiently and has disappeared, and all this took place without any genetic counseling and I think this is a quite interesting example of a system which without planning worked in an exemplary fashion in most countries, but that is my opinion: I would like to see genetics integrated rather than segregated.

Epstein: I think actually we are not as far apart as you think, because the frame of what I am advancing within the American system essentially is to keep genetic counseling in medicine. I think Dr. Motulsky would probably talk about it more, but we see a tendency for people to get very much involved in genetic matters completely apart from medicine and even not have medically trained people involved, and this is something we have been concerned with. Secondly, we have not yet attained the situation which, I agree with you, would be very desirable, of having the practising physicians, the pediatricians, and so on, handle the more common multifactorial conditions, for instance Down's syndrome, really the common bread and butter of the counseling problems. This is a goal that I have set forth. This type of centralized system that we talked about has a major problem, which is that we do not have the manpower to go around. It is unlikely that we will have the manpower in genetic counseling to cover certainly our population for many years to come. In an attempt to respond to that lack of manpower and at the same time to provide access of the patient to counseling and to provide them with a good level of counseling, we have come to try to have centralized systems such as we are dealing with. I think you have to keep in mind that a country of say, the size of England and Scotland combined, is not much bigger than the state of California in its land mass. And yet the population size you have in England and the number of those involved in genetic matters is vastly in excess of what we have in California. So we do have different problems of distribution.

One further point: the use of paramedical personnel. That problem really derives from the fact that we do not have enough people medically trained in the area of genetics or genetically trained in the area of medicine. This is why I have stressed the psychological aspects of the counseling, which really require a lot of time. We try to free our physicians at the point where the diagnostic and the basic genetic work is done. I think this is a healthy trend wherever it is done, because I think that even in England, as the demand for the services becomes greater, you eventually will saturate your capacity to deliver them. We are talking about the use of paramedical people – in the U.S. we speak of affiliated health personnel – but implicit in all of what I am saying there is actually a desire to keep genetic counseling in medicine rather than have it go out.

Mrs. Hagemeyer: What is the cost of genetic services in San Francisco, and who pays for it?

Epstein: The cost, if you calculate it out, is approximately $100 per patient. It is paid for by a combination of Governmental sources, research funds, a whole melange of funding mechanisms, all of which are basically unsatisfactory and unstable, and in the U.S. we are beginning to see movements, on a statewide basis to a national level, to put these support mechanisms on a more reasonable basis. Granting from either federal funds from the Government or from private agencies tends to be fairly constant in its amount, but though I hate to say so, we have inflation in the U.S. and our ability to support these types of service is being eroded. At the same time, in many areas the private insurance companies, which handle a lot of the payment for medical services, do not recognize genetic counseling as a valid item; in medical terms it is all right if your appendix is cut out, but it is no good being counseled. In the area of prenatal diagnosis, for example, we can get paid for doing the amniocentesis because it is in the book as a a legitimate obstetrical expense, but we cannot get paid for doing the chromosome analysis, because that is not listed in the book.

A lot of counseling can be done at a very reasonable price if it is handled on an efficient basis.

Anders: I wonder if you have a training program for counselors?

Epstein: I could ask what you mean by counselors. We have really two kinds of training programs now in the U.S. We have training programs for medical geneticists and Dr. Motulsky, for example, has one of the major training programs in this field in the U.S. These programs have gone through several stages. I think we have seen that in the past these programs were intended for people in medical genetics and genetic counseling who were originally trained in other areas of medicine. We are now seeing programs for newer groups with less training in other fields. They may have written a specialty thesis, say in internal medicine or in pediatrics, but are not sub-specialist in some field; they are now making medical genetics in a sense a subspecialty, and I think there are even some who will not be specialists in either field and essentially will become specialists in medical genetics. These types of training programs exist scattered around the country. There are essentially fellowship programs similar to what we have for other postgraduate medical training: apprentice type systems. We also have a few training programs in the U.S. for these other types of ancillary health people. They train people in basic genetics and in techniques of counseling and interviewing and the rest. Unfortunately, the problem with these training programs is that the functioning genetic counseling groups often do not have enough money to hire their graduates.

PROBLEMS OF SCREENING FOR GENETIC DISEASE*

A. G. MOTULSKY

Screening for genetic disease is done both to identify patients for treatment or prevention of a genetic disease which will cause serious harm, and to detect carrier states or predispositions which may lead to possible disease in the children of the predisposed. Screening programs in genetic diseases are sometimes also carried out to obtain incidence or prevalence data for scientific and public health reasons.

Population-wide screening for service rather than for research purposes should only be recommended a) when a disease or carrier state can be clearly defined, b) when reliable tests for detection are available, c) when proven treatment or preventive schemes exist, d) when full genetic services including genetic counseling and implementation of reproductive alternatives (such as amniocentesis) can be provided. A full discussion of the current state of genetic screening has been published (1).

SCREENING FOR TREATMENT AND PREVENTION

Phenylketonuria (2, 3). This autosomal recessive disease causes severe mental retardation since high phenylalanine levels caused by phenylalanine hydroxylase deficiency damage the brain. Blood phenylalanine levels are assayed by microbial inhibition techniques. Testing at 5-7 days of life is optimal for detection since some infants may not have elevated phenylalanine levels until that time. Phenylalanine-free diets when started early in life prevent mental retardation. Treatment can be discontinued at the age of 6-7 years. The frequency of the disease is 1/10,000-1/15,000 in Caucasian populations.

Follow-up of potentially affected infants requires good collaboration of biochemists, pediatricians, and nutrition specialists. Centralization or re-

* This work was supported by NIH grant GM 15253.

gionalization of laboratory facilities is strongly recommended. Hyperphenyl-alaninemia not associated with mental retardation occurs at rates somewhat lower than true phenylketonuria and does not require treatment. 'False positive' screening tests do occur and need to be fully worked out to prevent inclusion of infants without phenylketonuria in potentially harmful treatment regimens.

Girls with phenylketonuria need to be carefully followed and instructed about their disease since their high phenylalanine levels will injure the brain of their heterozygote fetuses in utero and produce mental retardation unless the phenylalanine-free diet is reinstituted (4).

The validity of phenylketonuria screening programs cannot be measured by simplistic cost-benefit analyses with emphasis on economics alone. Such analyses do not usually consider that phenylketonuria patients only comprise 1% of residents in mental retardation hospitals. Disappearance of phenylketonuria patients following screening only reduces the costs of such hospitals by a small margin (5).

Inborn errors of metabolism other than phenylketonuria (6). Using the same blood specimen collected for phenylketonuria testing, many other inborn errors can be tested for at birth. These include diseases such as homocystinuria, maple syrup urine disease, galactosemia, and others. These diseases are usually rarer than phenylketonuria – and are found in 1/75,000-1/200,000 infants. Treatment is much less standardized than for phenylketonuria and some are untreatable. Some inborn errors such as histidinemia were thought to cause disease but turned out to be innocuous variants. It is possible to add tests for many of these rare metabolic diseases to the phenylketonuria testing program. Previous experience with phenylketonuria and other genetic diseases suggest that many 'false positive' tests will be obtained for each disease and that for each disease genetic heterogeneity is likely. Additional tests for different diseases therefore will increase the logistical problems of the screening program. Even though testing for a variety of inborn errors may be inexpensive and simple in the laboratory, planners of screening programs must be prepared for recall of many babies who ultimately will turn out to be normal.

Down's syndrome (see 7 for references). The frequency of Down's syndrome increases sharply with advancing maternal age. The risk for a woman of 40 years or older to have an affected child is around 1%. Amniocentesis at the beginning of the second trimester of pregnancy can diagnose Down's syndrome by chromosome study. It has therefore been recommended that this procedure be made available to all mothers above 38-40 years of age.

If Down's syndrome is diagnosed, the option of selective abortion can be offered. Amniocentesis has proven to be a safe procedure for mother and fetus. The possibility of the rare complications of treatable maternal bleeding or infection or fetal needle marks is outweighed by the risk of severe untreatable mental retardation of Down's syndrome.

At the present time, facilities for a program which screens *all* women at risk do not exist in any country. The development of such programs has a high priority for public health since almost 50% of all cases of Down's syndrome are born to mothers above 38 years of age. Problems of abortion of affected fetuses raise religious and ethical problems for many parents and need to be handled on an individual basis. The final decision regarding abortion must be left to the parents but every parent-at-risk should be told about the option of amniocentesis. Laws concerning abortion of affected fetuses are changing rapidly in many countries.

Tay-Sachs disease (8). Tay-Sachs disease is a progressive neurologic disease leading to gross mental and physical deterioration and death between the ages of 3-6 years. The condition is an autosomal recessive trait and has a frequency of about 1/4000 in Jews of Ashkenazi (Eastern-European) origin. This frequency implies that 3-4% of such Jews are heterozygote (unaffected) carriers. Carriers can be identified by demonstrating a relative deficiency of the enzyme hexosaminidase A. Affected fetuses can be distinguished from carrier-heterozygote and unaffected fetuses by appropriate enzyme assays on amniotic fluid cells.

Parents with an affected child or parents who are both heterozygote but usually do not know that they are carriers, have a 25% chance of a child with Tay-Sachs disease. Amniocentesis allows determination of fetal hexosaminidase status. Selective abortion of affected fetuses makes it possible for such parents to have normal children. Population screening for Tay-Sachs disease can identify carrier x carrier matings *before* an affected child is born and has been initiated among the Jewish population of several U.S. cities. At the present time most of these programs are carried out under the auspices of community organizations rather than under the health departments. Even with an in Jews relatively common disorder such as Tay-Sachs disease, only one out of every 1000 matings between Ashkenazi Jews are at risk.

Sickle cell and β-thalassemia (see 9-12 for references). The sickle cell trait is common among many populations of African origin. Thus, 8% of U.S. blacks carry the trait. The trait itself appears to be harmless. Mating of trait x trait persons will cause sickle cell anemia in 25% of their children. Sickle cell anemia is associated with moderate to severe hemolytic anemia and periodic joint and abdominal pain. Approximately one-half of all patients with sickle cell anemia are said to have died by the age of 20 years in the U.S.

The sickle cell trait can be easily detected by simple electrophoretic methods. Other hemoglobinopathy traits such as Hb C and β-thalassemia are also common in U.S. black populations and occur with frequencies of 2-3% and 0.5-1%, respectively (13). Compound heterozygotes such as Hb S-C and Hb S-β-thalassemia are less severely affected than patients with sickle cell anemia. β-Thalassemia trait is common in some Greek and Southern Italian communities as well as in S.E. Asia. The homozygous state for β-thalassemia causes severe anemia with early mortality unless such patients are transfused frequently.

Screening for the sickling trait was initiated in many cities of the United States. Unfortunately, screening programs frequently were not accompanied by sufficient education and counseling. Sickle cell trait carriers often thought that they were ill or predisposed to develop sickle cell anemia. The medical profession also was not well informed regarding the usual absence of medical implications of the sickling trait. Stigmatization of sickle cell carriers for insurance and occupational purposes sometimes resulted. Programs were established indiscriminately and young children and old persons beyond the reproductive period were tested. The distinction of testing for a *disease* such as sickle cell anemia which could not be treated and testing for the *trait* for which reproductive advice only could be given was often not made. An evaluative study in a community in Greece where sickling was common showed social stigmatization but no effects in reduction of sickling trait x sickling trait matings (14).

Screening for sickling and/or thalassemia therefore needs further study and assessment. In the future, intrauterine diagnosis for the hemoglobino-pathies may become more practical (15-17). Such a procedure requires aspiration of fetal blood from the umbilical vein under direct vision or following placental puncture preceded by altrasound localization. Subsequently radioactive assays of the extent of Hb β chain synthesis for thalassemia diagnosis and of Hb β^s synthesis for diagnosis of sickle cell anemia can be performed. More widespread application of such intrauterine techniques can justify screening programs, since decisions regarding choice of marriage partner based on hemoglobin type or preclusion of children in trait x trait matings need no longer be considered if selective abortion of affected fetuses is acceptable. This mode of prevention provides fewer decisional difficulties for parents of the lethal thalassemia major than for parents of the less severe sickle cell anemia.

Pharmacogenetic disorders. G6PD deficiency of the red cell is a common trait among populations of tropical and subtropical origin (18). The defect is X-linked and is harmless unless certain drugs are administered or fava beans are eaten when hemolysis may occur. Different types of G6PD deficiency occur. The African type is less severe than the Mediterranean type. Screening of all hospitalized patients who may receive potentially hemolytic drugs would appear appropriate but is rarely performed.

Pseudocholinesterase variation makes for an abnormal pseudocholin-esterase molecule (19). One in 3000 Caucasians is homozygous for an atypical type of pseudocholinesterase and is unable to hydrolyze the muscle relaxant suxamethonium – a commonly used drug during anesthesia induction. Prolonged apnea results in affected homozygotes and requires artificial respiration. Screening tests for the abnormal enzyme are available but are usually not used prior to anesthesia (20).

RESEARCH OF OTHER SCREENING PROGRAMS

A variety of screening programs for genetic diseases are under investigation. These include amniotic fluid screening for α-fetoprotein, a substance which is elevated in spina bifida and related disorders (21). Retrospective screening by amniocentesis in women who had an affected child and therefore have a 3-4% chance of recurrence could identify affected fetuses for possible selective abortion. The total impact on the frequency of these disorders would be small. The possibilities of screening *all* pregnant women with serum α-fetoprotein determinations are under study to identify those who may carry affected babies (22, 23). The impact of this approach would be considerable.

Screening for α-antitrypsin deficiency will identify patients at risk to develop premature chronic obstructive pulmonary disease (24). No preventive treatment is available as yet.

Screening for the hyperlipidemias (25) is under active investigation. Several genetic diseases affecting lipid metabolism predispose to premature myocardial infarction. Unfortunately, apart from cholesterol and triglyceride levels we lack specific markers for these diseases and extensive family studies are required before a definite diagnosis of a genetic disorder can be made. Population screening of cord bloods cannot be recommended until better tests to identify those at high risk can be found. Similarly, existing dietary and drug regimens have not yet been proven to reduce the chance of heart attacks. More investigations are therefore required. Nevertheless, screening of family members of affected patients appears worthwhile.

Carriers for cystic fibrosis cannot yet be detected reliably. If such a test becomes available (and this might be the case within the next 5 years) and if fetuses with the disease can be diagnosed, widespread screening programs are likely to be established for this common disease (1/2000 in populations of European origin).

It may even become possible to detect those persons at risk to develop cancer of the lung from smoking. There are suggestions that the level of the enzyme aryl hydrocarbon hydroxylase which transforms polycyclic hydrocarbons to epoxides may be elevated in those persons who are likely to develop lung cancer (26).

In conclusion, screening for genetic diseases or carrier states is possible in several conditions. At the present time, only screening for phenylketonuria can be recommended as a service procedure. Screening for genetic diseases raises new problems in public health and considerably more assessment of existing programs is needed.

REFERENCES

1. *Genetic Screening. Programs, Principles, and Research.* Committee for the Study of Inborn Errors of Metabolism, Division of Medical Sciences, Assembly of Life Sciences, National Research Council. Washington, D.C., National Academy of Sciences (1975).
2. Knox, W. E., Phenylketonuria. In: Stanbury, J. B., J. B. Wijngaarden and D. S. Fredrickson (eds.), *The metabolic basis of inherited disease.* 3rd ed. McGraw-Hill, New York 1972. pp. 266-295.
3. Holtzman, N. A., Screening for phenylketonuria and its problems. In: A. G. Motulsky and W. Lenz (eds.), *Birth defects. Proceedings of the Fourth International Conference,* Vienna, September 1973. Amsterdam: Excerpta Medica 1974. pp. 263-267.
4. Maternal phenylketonuria. *Amer. Coll. Obstet. Gynecol. Tech. Bull.* No. 25, December 1973.
5. Motulsky, A. G., Brave new world? Current approaches to prevention, treatment, and research of genetic diseases raise ethical issues. *Science* 185, 653-663 (1974).
6. Levy, H. L., Genetic screening. *Adv. Hum. Genet.* 4, 1-104 (1973).
7. Milunsky, A., *The Prenatal Diagnosis of Hereditary Disorders.* Charles C. Thomas, Springfield 1973.
8. Kaback, M. M., R. S. Zeiger, L. S. Reynolds and M. Sonneborn, Approaches to the prevention and control of Tay-Sachs disease. *Prog. Med. Genet.* (in press).
9. Motulsky, A. G., Screening for sickle cell hemoglobinopathy and thalassemia. *Israel J. Med. Sci.* 9, 1341-1349 (1973).
10. Whitten, C. F. and J. Fischoff, Psychosocial effects of sickle cell disease. *Arch. Intern. Med.* 133, 681-689 (1974).
11. Gaston, M., Screening for sickle cell disease. *So. Med. J.* 67, 257-258 (1974).
12. Rutkow, I. M. and J. M. Lipton, Some negative aspects of state health departments' policies related to screening for sickle cell anemia. *Amer. J. Publ. Health* 64, 217-221 (1974).

13. Motulsky, A. G., Frequency of sickling disorders in U. S. blacks. *N. Engl. J. Med.* 288, 31-33 (1973).
14. Stamatoyannopoulos, G., Problems of screening and counseling in the hemoglobinopathies. In: A. G. Motulsky and W. Lenz (eds.), Fourth International Conference on Birth Defects, Vienna, September 1973. Abstracts of Papers. International Congress Series No. 297. Amsterdam: Excerpta Medica Foundation 1974. pp. 14-15.
15. Kan, Y. W., A. M. Dozy, B. P. Alter, F. D. Frigoletto and D. G. Nathan, Detection of the sickle gene in the human fetus. Potential for intrauterine diagnosis of sickle-cell anemia. *N. Engl. J. Med.* 287, 1-5 (1972).
16. Hobbins, J. C. and M. J. Mahoney, In utero diagnosis of hemoglobinopathies. *N. Engl. J. Med.* 290, 1065-1067 (1974).
17. Chang, H., J. C. Hobbins, G. Cividalli, F. D. Frigoletto, M. J. Mahoney, Y. W. Kan and D. G. Nathan, In utero diagnosis of hemoglobinopathies. Hemoglobin synthesis in fetal red cells. *N. Engl. J. Med.* 290, 1067-1068 (1974).
18. Motulsky, A. G., Hemolysis in glucose-6-phosphate dehydrogenase deficiency. *Fed. Proc.* 31, 1286-1292 (1972).
19. Motulsky, A. G. and A. Morrow, A typical cholinesterase gene $E_1{}^a$: Rarity in Negroes and most Orientals. *Science* 159, 202-203 (1968).
19. Motulsky, A. G. and A. C. Morrow, Atypical cholinesterase gene $E_1{}^a$: Rarity in Negroes and most Orientals. *Science* 159, 202-203 (1968).
20. Morrow, A. C. and A. G. Motulsky, Rapid screening method for the common atypical pseudocholinesterase variant. *J. Lab. & Clin. Med.* 71, 350-356 (1968).
21. Milunsky, A. and E. Alpert, The value of alpha-fetoprotein in the prenatal diagnosis of neural tube defects. *J. Pediat.* 84, 889-892 (1974).
22. Seller, M. J., J. D. Singer, T. M. Coltart and S. Campbell, Maternal serum – alpha-fetoprotein levels and prenatal diagnosis of neural tube defects. *Lancet* I, 428-429 (1974).
23. Harris, R., R. G. Jennison, A. J. Barson, K. M. Laurence, E. Ruoslahti and M. Seppala, Comparison of amniotic-fluid and maternal serum alpha-fetoprotein levels in the early antenatal diagnosis of spina bifida and anencephaly. *Lancet* I, 429-433 (1974).
24. Kueppers, F. and L. F. Black, α_1-antitrypsin and its deficiency. *Am. Rev. Resp. Dis.* 110, 176 (1974).
25. Motulsky, A. G. and H. Boman, Screening for the hyperlipidemias. In: *The prevention of genetic disease and mental retardation.* Milunsky, A. (ed.) Saunders, Philadelphia 1975.
26. Kellerman, G., C. R. Shaw and M. Luyter-Kellerman, Aryl hydrocarbon hydroxylase inducibility and bronchogenic carcinoma. *N. Engl. J. Med.* 289, 934-937 (1973).

DISCUSSION

PAPER OF A.G. MOTULSKY

de Jong: Did you study the hyperlipoproteinemias, viewed in the light of Fredrickson's hypercholesterolemia typing (4 or 5 types)?

Motulsky: Yes, we did, and we feel that while this type of subdivision has been pushed a lot it really is of no practical use. We feel that you can get just as much with measurements of fasting triglycerides and cholesterol. I think that there are many other groups now having similar experiences, so that the important thing to remember is that the lipoprotein phenotype is not a genetic type at all. The lipoprotein phenotypes are very far removed from what genes are doing. They can change in the same individual, and are not as easy to work with as initially was thought.

van Gemund: May I assume that recruits for the U.S. army are screened by the Army Medical Corps for sickle cell carriership and if so is the serviceman informed about the results?

Motulsky: There has been lots of discussion on what the armed forces should do about the sickling problem. There were suggestions that the sickling trait may cause problems under very unusual circumstances. On that basis it was suggested that every soldier had to be tested for this, and if he has a sickle trait he should be rejected service. However, the medical pathological effects are very unusual, and it would do grave injustice to thousands of people if they were to be rejected or excluded from the army, which means that they might be rejected for all kinds of occupations. So this is a very important issue, and most of those who have looked into the question have felt that if people want to be tested, they can be tested. If they are positive they need to be told about the genetic and medical consequences of the sickling trait; the latter are usually negligible.

ten Kate: You mentioned that you expect that a test for heterozygotes in cystic fibrosis will be available within five years. I wonder if this is not a bit speculative, and therefore I would like to ask you what kind of test you have in mind. In addition, there is the possibility of genetic heterogeneity in cystic fibrosis. You made a calculation that 400 matings are expected to give you one yield. I am wondering if there is really heterogeneity on more than one locus; if so, you might have to do much more work!

Motulsky: We do not know exactly what the test is going to be. The reason why I say it is going to be there within five years is that lots of laboratories are working on it. The celia inhibition factor seems to be something in the direction, but may not be the final answer. You know we have learned a lot about biochemistry and biochemical genetics in these systems, so that hopefully we will find out within five years, but I may be wrong. Concerning your second question, I agree that there may be heterogeneity. It is quite likely that even if you are only dealing with one locus there may be different mutational lesions in that locus, but then, even if you are a compound heterozygote for two such lesions, you might still have cystic fibrosis. If you have different loci, the situation might become more complicated.

Went: One of the reasons why you still might do amniocentesis in women over a certain age for detection of Down's syndrome, even in those who would not consider abortion, might be the relief of knowing that they are not carrying a Down's syndrome child. But it is possible that the child has an other defect, whether detectable or not.

Motulsky: Most of them cannot be detected, so it depends upon the right kind of counseling. It would be foolhardy to tell a woman you did the amniocentesis and everything is fine. All you can say is that we did not find a chromosome abnormality. If Down's syndrome was the indication and you know this was not found, this still does not rule out that all kind of other things can go wrong. I think a very careful discussion of all the things that can be found and those that cannot be found is extremely important before doing the amniocentesis, and since that needs to be done, good counseling needs to be done.

Eriksson: What do you think about the possibilities for detecting diabetes mellitus in families with a known diabetic history?

Motulsky: This is certainly such a common genetic disease that it would be nice if one could find out beforehand who is going to get it. But it would only be really useful if you could detect someone who is going to get diabetes five to ten years later if you could do something about it and prevent it. If you just found out that he is going to get it five years later, that might not help too much either. I think it is one of the great problems in this field.

Peña: At a certain point you mentioned to me that you would not advise a screening program in underdeveloped countries in view of the other urgent problems that have to be resolved. But I think that in South America, for example, where many women over the age of 40 bear children, a screening program for chromosomal abnormalities in this category seems justified.

Motulsky: When I talked about screening programs in underdeveloped countries I was thinking of inborn-error screening programs, where you have a frequency of 1 in 10,000 or something of that sort. Here again, logistics – the expense and all that goes into such a program – will make it very difficult to introduce them in such countries, but certainly it would be very nice if it were possible.

ten Kate: Concerning underdeveloped countries and screening for cystic fibrosis, I think we all know that cystic fibrosis, like phenylketonuria, has a different frequency in different races. At least, it is always said that cystic fibrosis is a frequent disorder in Caucasians. We really do not have any details about frequencies in underdeveloped Caucasian populations in for instance North Africa, the Near East, and India. So it may be that by screening these populations we might shed some light on the problem of why this disease is so frequent in Caucasian populations – whether the reason is racial or geographic.

Motulsky: But that is screening for research, to find out what it is all about; what we are talking of in this connection is screening to help people.

POPULATION EFFECTS OF GENETIC SCREENING

J. H. EDWARDS

Genetic disorders in man are conveniently divided into the chromosomal and the genic. The former are mainly sporadic, and associated with the inability to reproduce and uninfluenced by genetic screening, except in the obvious sense that they become rarer if aborted.

The main genic burden carried by man, and evident in clinical medicine, is that of recessive genetic disease. Dominant disorders are more readily catalogued and, to the philatelist of medicine, more numerous in their acknowledged variety, although not in the number of their victims. X-linked disorders, through the peculiar and incurable tragedy of muscular dystrophy, and the peculiar, and transiently curable, disorders of blood clotting, the haemophilias, or, in English, haemophilia and Christmas disease (Haemophilia B), are individually better known.

However, recessives are the commonest of the genic disorders, and it is these that I wish to discuss. As I am speaking with reference to Holland, a country close to Britain in the incidence of disease among its nativeborn population, I will restrict myself to the general problems of this population, and overlook the haemoglobin variants which impose peculiar opportunities for the conveying of advice through the ease and precision of heterozygote diagnosis.

In northern caucasians the commonest recessive disorder is clearly cystic fibrosis, with an incidence of about 1 in 2,000, a carrier frequency of about 1 in 20 and a gene frequency of about 1 in 40. The next commonest recessives are phenylketonuria, adrenogenital syndrome, and albinism, with frequencies of around 1 in 10,000 or less, and gene and heterozygote frequencies of the order of 1% to 2%.

If we enumerate all the disorders, and all their heterozygote proportions, we find that at least 50% of the population is a carrier of some potentially lethal, or severely disabling, allele. Less direct methods suggest that most of us are carriers for more than one or even more than two. However, the accountancy of clinical disorders is sufficiently precise to cast doubt on so onerous a genetic load.

Given this recessive burden we have the duty of attempting to pass on as little as possible to our descendants, and it is with this excellent and humane motive that applied human genetics must justify any practical application.

We may envisage the genic material of one generation as so many 'blots' or burdens, each representing a set of identical morbid alleles whose number is proportional to their area (fig. 1). The next generation is shown to the

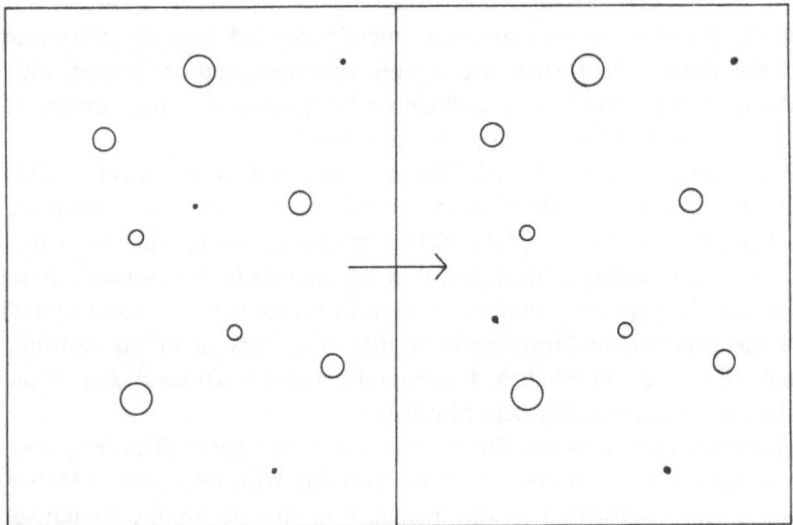

Fig. 1. Genetic load represented as lethal and detrimental alleles, which are conveyed from generation to generation with sampling variation, slight losses, and occasional novelties.

right. We may see that some very small ones are lost, and some new ones arise, and we may consider how such actions as are in the limited repertoire of clinical genetics (fig. 2) might reduce the burden borne by our descendants.

First, it is necessary to point out that natural loss arises from death, or, at least, death of the allele from non-reproduction, and that, since such an event only arises in the homozygous state, the number of deaths necessary to clear a population of 2N alleles is N individuals. If most people carry lethals, then the cost of clearance is at least of the same order as the population; that is, to rid Holland of genic disease, given unlimited diagnostic facilities, some ten-million or so non-births would have to be planned. Obviously, this is impractical, and it is necessary to live with the problem and to devote

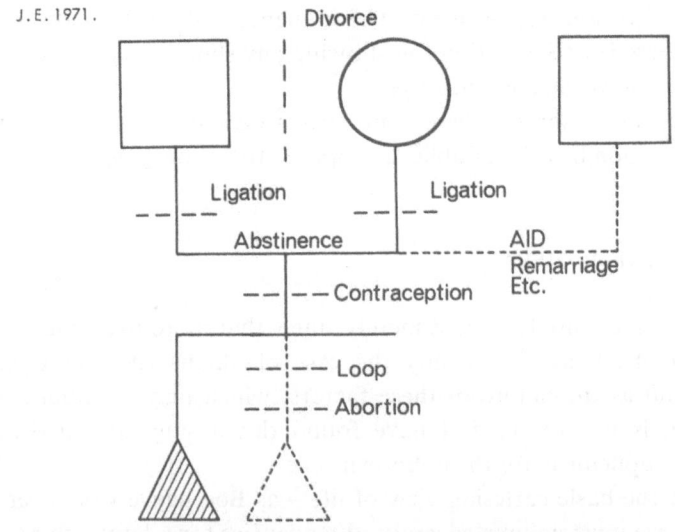

Options for artificial selection

Fig. 2. Diagram of options available in genetic counseling.

efforts to make it more tolerable, while considering the possibilities of a steady reduction.

It is often implied that the incidence of recessive disorders is maintained by mutations; in fact, this is probably true of the total, and new forms are continuously arising while the established forms are dying out. There is no reason to anticipate any focal stability – all that can be anticipated is an approximate balance involving the total frequency.

At present, in view of absence of any evidence to the contrary, as well as the sharp racial distribution, and the rapid growth of isolates in the past, we can assume all the recognized recessives are dying out with their hosts, and the effect of therapy, if successful, will be to stabilize their frequency, which is at present decreasing at a rate, per generation, approximating to the gene frequency.

Fetal diagnosis, followed by premature death, will have no effect on frequency of itself, although, if this increases the likelihood of a further birth, it will clearly reduce the decline in gene frequency, the reduction depending on the extent of such compensation. As affliction results from two abnormal alleles, neither of which would survive, and replacement by a non-homozygote with, on average, 4/3 abnormal alleles, which would survive, amniocentesis will have an effect intermediate between successful therapy and natural death without replacement. The influence will, in any case, be very slight, and there is no indication for allowing any short term decisions to be influenced by long term consequences.

In the recessive disorders there is no strong indication, or contra-indication, for any action based on public, as opposed to private good.

MULTIFACTORIAL DISEASE

This term is widely used; since it merely states that more than one factor is probably involved, as is evidently the case of all disorders of unknown aetiology, and as the nature of these factors, which may be inborn or environmental, is not specified, I have found this a singularly useless and unnecessary euphemism for the unknown.

If we take the basic cartesian view of life – as Boerhaave would certainly have done – we must assume generalized tendencies for relatives to resemble each other in health and disease, and, in consequence, for diseases to tend to run in families.

In the so-called multifactorial conditions we must suppose that the mean phenotype has evolved under selective pressures, and, under these pressures, there has been selection against both extremes. If we take the simple model of a diathesis, or a predisposition, as advanced by Hippocrates, then we can follow Pearson in giving this a numerical interpretation by truncation of a normal distribution. Obviously, if this minority was selected against through disease, or disability, or inadequate ability, or unacceptability for marriage, or through advice on genetical grounds, this would lead to the next generation having a different mean, and also a smaller scatter. In this model, since the distribution in the next generation would not be normal there would be difficulties in algebraic treatment.

It might seem that, as many disorders are related to the consequences of some underlying distribution, some discouragement of the reproductive potential of these minorities might benefit them by reducing the numbers of their afflicted children and might also benefit other peoples' descendants by reducing the incidence of disease in the future. In practice, little can be done; any change in the mean or variance of the underlying distribution will reduce the variability of the population, and, while a reduction in variability in relation to some unconditionally harmful alleles may be welcome, any overall reduction in variability will be so unpredictable in its consequences that these are as likely to be disadvantageous as advantageous.

In general clinical consequences only arise at one end of these distributions. An excess of detachment from the environment leads to schizophrenia; a failure of any capacity of detachment leading to a slavish dependance on reality, a condition more appropriate to computers than to people, leads to no clinical problem.

Too much cholesterol, uric acid, or glucose in the blood leads to clinical problems: the consequences of too little are hardly known, largely due to lack of study, but these substances have not evolved to give employment to physicians or geneticists, they are the stuff of life, and too little must, on an evolutionary basis, be as serious as too much. We have no rationale for attempting to influence the reproductive behaviour of such 'deviants'. Nor, fortunately, is there much indication for any advice in the private situation of individuals wishing healthy children. The recurrence risks for disorders of unknown aetiology are uniformly low – usually around 3% – so that some 95% of cases are the first in the family to be afflicted. Any reduction of fertility after affliction is inefficient, in that some thirty normal non-births is the cost of one afflicted non-birth, an efficiency of about 3%, and ineffective, in that some only 5% or so of cases follow a previous case.

Elaborate predictive schemes using implicit regression procedures have been developed to give exact risks for various relationships, but a regression line can be no better than the points on which it feeds, and, since the points must be specified, it may as well be used. If the recurrence risk is observed to be, for example, 7/156, then no estimate based on a regression line can improve on this estimate: nor is there any reason to suppose extrapolation to more distant relationships any more secure. Fortunately, there is little demand for exact values of low risks, for, in the perspective of total risk, disorders of unknown aetiology in second or third degree relatives are of little consequence.

This may seem a very hopeless approach; should we not be able to influence reproduction so as to maximise the health of our descendants. Unfortunately, selection, either by disease or by advice, can but modulate the total morbidity, since we must all die, and will mostly die from common disorders.

No doubt, rare disorders with predictable inheritance will be resolved and identified. A proportion of psychotics have Huntington's chorea; a proportion of hypertensives have familial chromatin tumours; a proportion of epileptics have epiloia; and a proportion of colonic tumours are due to multiple polyposis. But in all these cases we are dealing with small proportions, and the nature of the familial intensity makes it unlikely that detailed studies will more than double the proportion of strongly familial conditions.

In the single-locus disorders we have private advantages in advice, in that many parents at high risk may wish to respond to such advice: the consequences to the population are small, though not necessarily beneficial. In the disorders not related to a single locus there is neither a private nor a public advantage in advice, and any influence on behaviour from counseling is so slight, so inefficient, and so ineffective, that it would seem unwise for unsolicited advice to be given.

DISCUSSION

PAPER OF J.H. EDWARDS

Motulsky: I tend to agree with you, but there are some ideas I would like to hear your comments on. I agree with you that it is certainly easier to understand the mechanism underlying chromosomal errors and single gene defects, but yet, as you stated, the large majority of the diseases we have to deal with in public health are of the sort that you talked about, and there is a genetic background of the kind that you alluded to. On the other hand, I think that a lot of optimism is justified in the sense that since genetic factors are involved, these genetic factors may not be as complex as you suggested. In hypertension or diabetes there may in fact be relatively few genes involved. And just as we have understood Tay-Sachs disease or phenylketonuria, the time may be very near in which it will become possible to isolate the major genes that contribute to this kind of variation.

I think it is dangerous to say: well, here are single genes or chromosomal diseases; on the other hand, we have the complex diseases. However, the complexity just means that the genes interacting in this complexity ultimately are not going to be different from the single genes, and if it becomes possible to work out these single genes, then these conditions too will become simple. The interactions of the major genes can be rather complex, but still they are not mystical and they could be worked out, similarly to what is now possible with the single gene diseases. Furthermore, I think there are also some hints from biochemical genetics in which direction one might go, but I feel, and I think others feel with me, that since there are so many polymorphisms around, it is quite possible that these polymorphic genes in search of something, may in fact be part of this genetic background and that some of the polymorphisms may be tied up with some of these common diseases. You know, there are already hints for the HLA and the immune response systems, in which simple genes are involved. So I think the dichotomy you set out between simplicity and complexity may not be as acute, and may in fact soon be solved.

Edwards: Accepted that you can get these prediction factors. Take the locus of

HLA, there again one can say that with a number of diseases, e.g. gluten sensitivity, you can divide the population into various groups (just as you could with the postulated enzyme on smoking and so on) in which the liability to disease is 1 in 4 to about 1 in 16. I think the ratio is about 16 to 1 for gluten sensitivity and then you have a locus which determines whether one can catabolize or accept a gluten, in the same way as your skin can be pigmented. There are people whose response to an exposure to sunlight is based on very simple genetic mechanisms. There are people with red hair and so on who have a very bad response to sunlight and people who are dark haired who actually enjoy it. I am not doubting that such a simple genetic mechanism will produce these very big effects but I cannot accept these examples. I can accept that any of them will have executive action, I mean what will you actually do when you HLA-type someone and that person chooses a spouse with a different HLA-type, do you put them on a bread-free diet before they have symptoms?

Smoking is a dangerous occupation for the whole population. Particularly smoking in pregnancy has more effect than all the amniocenteses you can do in the whole country. So these are very big effects, which are well understood, and it seems to me that smoking has to be accepted as a particularly hazardous procedure under certain conditions, as in pregnancy. It is a poor sort of tactics to say: well, it is really hereditary, smoking, and you just have to choose your genes! I think that the population has to be controlled and I think that in a starving world it is wrong to have large parts of the arable land turning out things which are rather purely toxic, like tobacco, or rather mildly toxic, like sugar. These are major political issues in comparison with, for example, the gluten sensitivity.

I suppose you could pick up the celiac people who have difficulties with bread, but I cannot see that it would be reasonable to breed a race of bread-eaters by counseling with special techniques. I think that among the hypertensives, there are few who would be picked out on the basis of a single gene defect.

Motulsky: To take hypertension, you accept – I do not fully accept it but there is probably some truth to it – that you should treat hypertension with antihypertensive drugs. This delays some of the complications of hypertension. If, however, you apply a scheme for studying families of index cases who have hypertension, you will find more in that group.

Edwards: So what do you do, I mean except make them eat less?

Motulsky: Eat less and give drugs in this case.

Edwards: Yes, and give drugs, yes.

Motulsky: There is some evidence, from rather large-scale studies, that using antihypertensive medication in moderate hypertension cuts down on the mortality and morbidity of hypertension. Now as I said – but I do not 100% accept it – I think there may be different types of hypertension and perhaps some respond to drugs and others do not. You can identify a group that in fact does have a shortened life expectancy and will respond to drugs; you know here is one helpful way of finding out that chemical type, which occurs in certain families, and do something about it, so I think one does not need to be as pessimistic as you are.

Edwards: I am not pessimistic at all; I thought I was being rather optimistic and think there is no problem with hypertension, I do not see any. I think there is no doubt that people – lots of people – are greatly improved if you put them on antihypertensive drugs; they can see again, for example; they stop having fits. There does not seem to be any doubt that the drugs work at high levels, but is there any point in being picked up for hypertension with any device except a sphygmomanometer? Is there anybody to say this person is going to have high blood pressure, therefore we should give treatment? That would be a minority view for most physicans; they would wait for the blood pressure. So you might screen a population with the sphygmomanometer annually or every five years, which in fact is often done for insurances. But what I cannot quite see is how you can execute this information by childhood screening, for example of specific groups, because they have to wait to get the hypertension.

Motulsky: Yes, but the point I would want to make is that to measure the blood pressure might make us understand what genes are doing, and there may be subgroups of people with hypertension you could subdefine through rennin measurements or some chemical measurements. There may be a different gene which responds much better to your treatment than others do.

Veltkamp: Did you find high blood pressure in children whose parents have high blood pressure? Normal values for children are known at present, so you could screen at an early age.

Edwards: The trouble with blood pressure is that we simply do not know what would be the optimal level to be stabilized in a population, and whether there is evidence of any influence it has on the physical or intellectual achievements. Little is known about the dynamic group of people with high blood pressure who rush all over the place, always getting coronaries. I think there must be some basis for this, and one does not really know what happens. I mean you need sugar, you need cholesterol, and you need a driving force and these are main requirements for the brain. The brain cannot control anything, it just has to take what comes up the carotid, so if you are going to stop things going up, the brain will get reduced concentrations. On a population scale you have to know what the optimal blood pressure of a population is and what we were actually discussing was genetic screening. I cannot see any practical situation in which someone with these high levels should be discouraged from reproducing on those grounds. There are subgroups with exotic conditions, pheochromocytoma or something, and you can tell them there is a very high risk of hypertension and you can look at their children, and so on. But I was thinking just of the hypertensives in general; hypertension is an unpleasant condition, it leads to an early but not usually particularly unpleasant death, and what can you do about it, I mean if you exclude therapy? I cannot see this as a genetic problem – hypertension not any more than schizophrenia. I can see that it is a very big problem and that society has the need to put some of its resources into treatment and, in cases of schizophrenia, custodial care, but I cannot see that there is any justification for influencing someone else's reproductive behaviour on the grounds of any of these conditions which are not understood. I can see that with Huntington's chorea, for example, one should exert such influence. It is difficult to see that anybody with this condition is not an infected member of the population in just the same way as somebody with typhoid is. But are there any conditions under which you would advise people about reproduction on the basis of their blood pressure?

Motulsky: Not their blood pressure; but suppose that you have two parents both of whom have schizophrenia and they ask your advice. The risk is very high for their children. They might benefit from that advice and have fewer children.

Edwards: Yes, but this is a hypothetical situation. I mean, schizophrenics, like mental defectives, would not ask advice. So how do you counsel people who cannot understand? By the way, in your large experience, which is very large, have you ever had two schizophrenics come to you?

Motulsky: Only one.

Edwards: Oh, one.

Motulsky: But in my practice I do not see many psychiatric patients.

Edwards: What I mean is, this is the standard thing like whether you are driving along or you have to run into a Leonardo da Vinci or a busqueue. I mean there are all these standard moral problems, but I have never encountered this problem, two schizophrenics wanting advice. This hypothetical problem will not affect the numbers of schizophrenics. I just do not see in practice how you can do that except by enforcement and I think enforcement obviously creates bigger problems than anything else. Besides, schizophrenics are the most uncounselable group of people; if they are afraid of ghosts, they do not take your advice even if you are an experienced psychiatrist.

PANEL DISCUSSION:
ETHICAL ASPECTS OF PREVENTION

de Froe: The physician acts on the basis of his examination and of the inter-
pretations of his findings; he gives advice and thus intervenes in human life. The
actions of the human geneticist reach even further. He can have a great influence on
a family, within a marriage, within a human life. He makes decisions, acts on the
basis of a science, but it is not a science that coaches him in all aspects of what he
does: ethics forms a very important part of it. Compared to medicine, it is an
entirely different type of science, it is often very difficult to understand how an
ethicist reaches his point of view.

I thought it a good idea to let the ethicists on the panel give a short exposé of
the views they hold and how they arrive at their propositions.

Heering: I found it a fascinating challenge to come and take part in your meeting. You put ethics at the end and not at the beginning, but not because you want
ethics necessarily to have the last word. Ethics is not an absolute science; I may
quote Dr. Motulsky in this respect: 'Ethical systems are the products of the human
brain and lack an absolutist basis'. I believe that we should be very pleased that this
is recognized. I shall come back to the fact that ethics is a radical science, but not an
absolute one.

I am going to begin with a very ordinary question: How do you arrive at your
moral decisions? If I try to put myself in your position, I can do two things: I can
ask myself, first of all, what my motives are for my actions, and secondly, I can
try to place myself in the other person's position: what effect will my decisions
have on him? We consider ourselves powerful beings. We have a great deal of
power over the situation in which we live, power that we can use to do a lot of good
but also to do a lot of harm. All this makes it very necessary that we reflect on what
we do with our scientific abilities. We can talk to someone else. The first person we
would choose to talk to is probably someone who shares the same view of life as
we do. Or perhaps we prefer to talk to someone in particular no matter what his
view of life is but whom we expect to have insight and judgment and therefore to be
able to give a useful opinion.

We do not take a decision in isolation, nor can it depend upon individualistic
ethics. In this context I have four motives:

1. In the first instance, for every decision it is necessary to have proper information.
   Information concerning the disease, information concerning the person and his
   view of life.
2. The second motive I shall call 'ethos', that is, our moral attitude. This determines our basic motives.
3. The third motive is found in the social situation. You have to take into account
   how people think about such subjects as abortion or euthanasia.
4. And the last point you have to take into account is the anticipated outcome.

All these motives play an important role in decision-making. They explain why, for
example, two Roman Catholics adhering to the same 'ethos' nevertheless proceed

very differently in practice. On the other hand, Humanists and Protestants can start from a different 'ethos' but come to the same result.

Information alone is not sufficient; two persons receive the same information in different ways. The anticipated outcome is in itself not decisive either; we cannot act only pragmatically.

The final point in our decisions is the general wellbeing of the person concerned. The child should take first place in our decisions; in the second place come the parents, and lastly society. It is very difficult when we are confronted with defective life to decide whether one can speak of wellbeing. I am inclined to say, let us speak of prevention of suffering rather than promotion of wellbeing. When we talk about promotion of wellbeing we have a tendency to moralize, to create norms to which life is supposed to adhere.

Ethics is an auxiliary science which can help us to clarify our motives but does not give precise patterns according to which one should act. According to me, ethics does not give absolute certainties, but it does provide radical ones.

Beemer: I have been asked to say something about the question of who must decide with respect to the prevention of genetic defects. In the preface to this volume a double meaning is given to the prevention of inherited disorders, on the one hand prevention of birth of individuals with an inherited disorder and on the other hand prevention of the development of symptoms of disease in people having such a disorder.

Who takes part in the activities leading to prevention and the decisions following from them? The problems involved here concern the risk of having or not having a child, the possibilities for treatment, genetic research, sterilization, abortion, anticonception, and many others. Here, I should like to quote a theologian, Thomas Aquinas, who said: 'God has placed man in hands of his own counsel. Man makes provision for himself and for others as part of God's providence'. But even without subscribing to a religion, we can say that making provisions to prevent suffering is part of human dignity. If we accept that it is part of human dignity to make these provisions, then this prevention of suffering is a moral task for all of us. We must promote that people make their own decisions and we must strive, as far as possible, to agree on which decisions are good and which decisions are bad.

Now, to come back to the original question of who is entitled to take decisions in this question of genetic suffering, in my opinion there are three categories:

1. Those who are involved in procreation, i.e. potential parents;
2. Physicians and geneticists, who are experts in giving genetic advice and who work out the risks, and
3. Authorities who act on behalf of the community organized as a state.

With respect to the first category, the prevention of birth of individuals with hereditary diseases is in the last resort the decision of those who take part in this reproduction. They can only bear this responsibility if they are well informed. They have a right to good information, which is more than just telling them the chance for having a healthy or a defective child. The seriousness and the duration of any defect must also be explained in such a manner that they can consider these chances in relation to themselves and their family and also weigh these chances against the interests of the community.

The second category is formed by the physicians, or more specifically the geneticists, who act as advisers, experts; they can give parents information on the seriousness of the defect, they can estimate the chances of the risk involved. In some circumstances they must do this even if they have not been asked to do so. I believe that these experts should not have an independent position in this question of prevention of the birth of children with inherited diseases. However, they have their own responsibility if they have to initiate treatment. In counseling, if it is to go further than just giving information, we have to think of all of the standards current in society, current for the potential parents and for the counselors. You can give good advice only if you know what standards are important to the parents and what effect this has on their psyche. You have to know what is acceptable to them. In my opinion, objective criteria for acceptability or non-acceptability of risks cannot be formulated.

The third category comprises the authorities, who are concerned with two aspects: promotion of the wellbeing of individuals and promotion of the wellbeing of the society as a whole. The government should ensure that as much information is available as possible and necessary to enable the individuals to reach preventive decisions. Our society has the problem of population policy, particularly concerning the qualitative aspects. It is a fundamental question whether authorities have the right to prevent the birth of children in families with a high genetic risk.

The ethicist, in my view, is not entitled to take this type of decision. He can serve as adviser, to clarify the objectives and the values which individuals must take into consideration when they have to make such decisions.

Roscam Abbing: My principal point of view is primarily concerned with the interest of the child that has been or might be conceived. This brings me to the field of negative eugenics, which belongs to the realm of individual care. I shall not take into consideration the question of whether you can improve the state of the population as a whole; here, I shall restrict myself to the interests of and concern for the as yet unborn individual, so as to prevent extraordinary suffering. This is not only a question of sorrow and pain, but also of whether a person is equipped to carry out his task as a human being. I especially want to consider the prevention of the birth of children with a genetic disease. Once a child has been born, you must do what you can in terms of medical, surgical, or social treatment. The most delicate situation concerns the induced abortion. If you find from your prenatal examinations that there will be a really serious disease, then I consider that induced abortion is justified.

The main question is, however, whether people have the right to conceive a seriously disabled child. In this context they should consider – if necessary with the help of a genetic counselor – the following three points: the extent of the risk, the seriousness of the disease, and the extent of secondary effects. The extent of the risk includes some amount of uncertainty, but an evaluation seems possible. Consideration of the seriousness of the disease includes an evaluation of ethical, moral, and religious concepts. Mental defects weigh very heavily for me. If you are mentally healthy and physically handicapped, you can still have a splendid life to some extent. I find mental defect more serious, although it may be less painful. The secondary effects include stress on the parents and the rest of the family, and the care and expense which may have to be borne by society.

We must strive for a balance between all those who have to give counsel on these points. Each case is unique. If there is a very serious defect and a very high risk, then the question arises whether non-directive advice to the parents suffices. The previous speaker said rightly that the potential parents are the people who in the first instance bear the responsibility, and we must give them as much information as possible to enable them to make such a decision. The principal question is whether the authorities can continue to stand aside. I personally believe that proposals should come from society and notably from a group like the one present here today. If we say the parents have a right to information, this should include the need for registration of hereditary defects. With such registration, succeeding generations will have much more information at their disposal. I know there are problems associated with professional secrecy, but these should not interfere with registration and information. Giving information is the minimum we have to do; obligatory examination before marriage would be one of the next steps. At the moment, we now and again see individuals who really should not marry one another, or at least should not have a family. And at the moment, you can advise against it but you cannot prevent it. You can say that this is a very private matter and, certainly after Hitler's frightful practices during the war, people are frightened by the idea of any form of intervention. We have to be extremely careful on this point, but if we do not take any action there will be more victims. So I think that the authorities – democratically elected and controlled – should be able to go further than they do now, they should see to it that there are maximum facilities for providing information. They should see to it that examination before marriage is instituted, and as a consequence it should be possible to say you two people are not suitable for one another, at least if you intend to found a family. Sterilization could be one method, but of course there are other means. This is very dangerous ground but we must be realistic enough to tackle the problems. I will expressly say that we must not look at this problem as though it were a matter of severity or cruelty; it is a question of love and care for the unborn child. A child to be born should have maximum care under optimal conditions.

de Froe: We have had the general introduction. The ethicists have indicated not only who and how, but also what about. The situation is one in which we must have as much reliable information as possible and the decisions have to be geared to the future. We now have a basic approach to the way in which we should think about these questions, such as prevention, abortion, and euthanasia, and can proceed to the questions themselves.

Kortman: Roscam Abbing says that he proceeds from the point of view of the child, but according to me he proceeds from the point of view of society. I suppose you know the following quotation: 'Who with me as a Christian is convinced that man is created in relation to God, can never say that the life of someone who has this relation to God has no meaning. People who cannot be certain of their relation to God because of their mental deficiencies, can still have a relationship because God has a relation to them'; it comes from Roscam Abbing!

Roscam Abbing: I said the interest of the child, whereas you say that I was actually talking about the interest of society. Are these really two different concepts?

We as society should put the interest of the child, of the individual, first; do you agree with that?

Kortman: Yes, I do, but I deny that you did.

Roscam Abbing: Aha, I have the impression that you find two inconsistent points in my argumentation. Firstly, my starting point and the rest of my arguments; secondly, the contents of the citation and what I have been talking about. You might imagine this is not as inconsistent as you suggest, otherwise I should be a very scatterbrained person. I insist that everything turns around the interest of the child and I am sure you agree with me there.

We are talking about someone who is not born, or even has not been conceived. The interest of those not yet conceived is that they should not be conceived if one might expect conception to result in dramatic suffering and a terrible form of life. We concentrate so much on relieving minor burdens that it would be ridiculous not to prevent fundamental, enormous burdens. This is precisely the reason which makes me search for everything possible we can do to prevent the birth of such children.

The essential question is whether such a life is without sense. You quoted my words to the effect that 'the relation to God is fundamental'. I am consciously a Christian. Some, like me, speak of the conscious relation to God, others say conscious relation to the values of life, but always the word 'conscious' is used. And this is why, in my opinion, mental defects are the most difficult to accept. I made the restriction that even if we are not aware of a relation to God, it does not mean that God has no relation to us. But does this mean that we are not entitled to attempt to prevent such lives? Although we know that sickness can be enormously productive spiritually, we still do everything in our power to prevent it.

Kortman: You agree in principle with abortion and you are prepared to go further, even after birth. But is this in the interest of the child to be, since you have said there is a relation from God to the child? These points cannot be reconciled with one another. I think that you proceed from the point of view of the parents and society. Such a defective child probably does not suffer at all and at least suffers much less than a normal person during his whole life. Only the parents and society are going to have a hard time. The child itself from which you proceed – that child would be damaged by being robbed of its existence.

de Froe: May I interrupt? My point of view is that the parents and the doctor, discussing this question about the child who is not yet conceived or not yet born, also have a relation with God and it is from this relation that their decisions emanate.

Kortman: My next question is concerned with legislation. You talked about the nefarious practices of Hitler, but I think that we will come very close to those practices if the government is entitled to intervene in the intimate life of people and can even take action to prevent them from having children.

Roscam Abbing: If we were to approach such practices in any way it would be very serious indeed, but you must not spoil the discussion with associations to something that is really completely different. Hitler's intentions were totally different; for him it was not a question of limiting suffering, which is our only concern.

It is a very delicate question how far the authorities can go in interfering with the private life of a citizen. As far as I am concerned, I wonder if you realize how far the authorities have already penetrated into the private life of the individual, and I would say rightly. Children are forced to go to school. The authorities are also entitled to remove children from their parents. They are empowered to give vaccinations. All this has been accepted on the ground that the authorities are not only entitled but obliged to prevent asocial actions of citizens. The authorities have the right to put someone in jail. These things represent a considerable infringement on the liberty of the individual. Why then should we not take these preventive measures (i.e., prevent the conception or birth of disabled children), since this too is a service to the parents. We are preventing them from being guilty of irresponsible procreation. And of course they themselves would be burdened by having to bring up a heavily handicapped child,

Gebhardt: I understand you would like to have laws requiring medical investigation before marriage. How do you achieve the optimum of national wellbeing? Is it desirable, is it practicable? I have heard the statement that the net result of vaccination programs in countries where vaccination is compulsory is not markedly different from that in countries where it is not. To save lives, it would perhaps be much more useful to provide more traffic lights than to spend money on an expensive population examination. So I should like to know where you think the priorities are.

Roscam Abbing: One should not combat a good aim with a better one. It is quite possible that we should have more traffic lights, but that is another matter. Concerning your question (is it realizable, is it going to help?), I would refer to my proposition that the authorities ought to introduce legislation leading to such examinations for potential parents and making registration of inherited defects obligatory. But *only* if these measures will be effective and if the practical difficulties are not too great. You are evidently worried about these practical difficulties, but according to me they are not unsurmountable. There should be a national commission to study these problems, to which I think you should be appointed.

Koning: I want to say two things. First, I believe that the handicap is not terrible for the child, it is happy in its own surroundings. It is only a sad thing for the parents. Is it right that we should undertake steps to prevent the birth of such a child? Secondly, I think the question of legislation by the authorities should not be considered at all, because it would create such great problems in all layers of our society.

The parents' sense of responsibility will decrease rather than increase with the introduction of governmental action. Instead of that, we should use all available media (radio, TV, etc.) to give people more information on the subject.

de Froe: It has already been said twice that such a defective child need not suffer so much, but there are children who suffer their whole life only because they have a cleverer brother or sister. We are very poorly informed about the suffering of defective people. We cannot assume, certainly not without further study, that none of them suffer.

There are things which according to you should be achieved by propaganda and by information; for example, examination before marriage should be on a voluntary basis. But in my opinion it is important to let the state regulate this, because it only makes sense if everyone participates. Also the registration of genetic disease is only useful if it is complete.

Koning: My view is that we should not take the responsibility for the defective child away from the parents and put it into the hands of the authorities. Another matter is that via medical examination in families where handicapped children were born, you can show the parents that they have the responsibility in passing on hereditary disorders. These families have a personal responsibility for what they do, in their own interest and that of their descendents.

Heering: I am inclined to say that these problems are immense because counseling is so difficult. People have virtually no one with whom they can really talk. For example, women who go to the abortion team in Leiden have said that they have not been able to discuss their problems with anybody. They can hardly discuss them with the man who has fathered the child, even less so with close relatives, and usually these women do not have a pastor. All proposals to do away with measures originated by society are hypocritical, I think. Society cannot take away the burden of defective children from families; furthermore, the families usually cannot stand the burden. Society can only assist such families. We must be very thankful that social measures are taken so that people usually do not have to be in financial trouble, that there are sometimes institutions which accept these children. But it is simply not true that this removes the trouble and sorrow from the parents and the brothers and sisters of the defective child itself.

In the second place, I think that ethicists must not take such a high line here. It is not true that everone believes in God and therefore accepts his child as God's child. Certainly we also have to give medical help to people who do not have our so-called optimal moral basis, religious or otherwise. As regards what the authorities could do, I am rather more reserved than Roscam Abbing. I certainly recognize the problem, but I consider that the objections are greater than the advantages. Where do you end? I am inclined to accept that the authorities should make sterilization obligatory for people who are mentally deficient, but you, the medical profession, must decide who is mentally deficient.

I think it is frightfully important that medical men, ethicists, and other individuals should be prepared to help their fellow creatures as far as possible with advice, before the government has to step in.

Kortman: Mr. Heering referred to the obstetrician Sikkel and his team to whom women could come and talk. But Sikkel stopped this work quite soon, because he said they are not patients, they are clients. They should say what they want to have done and we are here to carry it out.

Mr. Roscam Abbing has stated that the law should be made in a very democratic manner. But he ignores the existence of a big group against whom we are discriminating here – the group of those who have not yet been born. They are also human beings, who have no possibility to speak for themselves.

de Froe: But Mr. Kortman, how would you let them speak?

Kortman: Yes, I quite agree that this is not possible, but that does not mean that they do not exist; they are complete human beings who have all the genes of their previous generation; they are ready to become fully equipped humans.

Bos: We are talking about prevention. But what I have missed so far is any reference to the task of the community in stimulating prevention. You have only talked about individuals and government. Prevention is quite possible at the moment. Anencephaly could be reduced to 10 % of the present level in The Netherlands if women would have their children between the ages of 20 and 30, and this applies to a great number of other conditions.

Beemer: You can advise a certain age for reproduction, and you relate this point to the task not of the government but of the community. The question is whether organizations which give information on health matters would provide such advice about limiting the period of reproduction. In the advantage you obtain by preventing a number of defective births – you consider this so important that you want to limit the reproductive age, which I see as a disadvantage in certain cases – you must weigh one point against the other.

I should just like to say that when the social or health organizations concerned can show what the effect of prevention is – limiting the reproductive age to between 20 and 30 years – then let them give such advice. The values which are at stake should be considered by the people themselves.

de Froe: For the sake of clarity, Mr. Kortman, in cases of proven anencephaly in the twelfth week, are you against induced abortion?

Kortman: In the case of anencephaly, too, I am against induced abortion. Anencephalics die at or shortly after birth.

de Froe: I do not think that everyone will agree with you on this point, but I wanted to hear you say it.

Delleman: I should like to ask Mr. Kortman if he takes into account that the woman who knows that she is bearing a child with anencephaly – what a terrible time that mother-to-be has? I think you are asking too much of the mother and are concentrating too much on the child in this case.

Kortman: The knowledge that you are carrying an anencephalic child is of course dreadful, and I really do not want to underestimate what the parents go through in this case. But on the other hand those who screen and determine genetic disorders in which the chance of a totally deformed child is great, should also realize what they are doing by telling the parents at such an early stage. But still the relation of God to the unborn child remains and there are numerous parents who would rather produce an anencephalic child than know that they have been guilty of their child being killed.

Hylkema: I am afraid that we are getting onto theoretical ground talking about reproduction between the ages of 20 and 30, because about 80 % of reproduction already takes place in this period. We should first talk about the problem of whether it makes sense to do genetic counseling and to identify those at risk, and furthermore whether abortion forms a solution for the problems we are concerned with.

Kuenen: I would like to make some remarks. As early as 1900, the gynaecologist Treub recognized the dilemma between interference of the authorities and the responsibility of the parents. My second remark is that if you introduce compulsory sterilization, people might move to neighbouring countries. All sorts of practical consequences can come from such compulsory measures. Lastly, I would like to mention an example of a boy of 19 who found out while in military service that he had hypercholesterolaemia. He knew whom he wanted to marry, that he could support a family, and that he had an illness which would not allow him to reach old age. He said to me, 'I can be just as happy living only 50 years instead of living

80 years. I just have to get things done more quickly. I want to marry now and I want to have children'.

Roscam Abbing: I should have hoped that the young man would have said, not 'I can be as happy in 50 as in 80 years', but 'If I die at the age of 50, my children will have had their father in the essential period for them'.

Roede: I have a comment, not a question. In my view of life, God does not play an important role and this does not interfere with my responsibilities. I know and feel that there are people who do not share my view of life, but I will not say that their philosophy is incorrect, nor will I interfere with their way of life, although they try to do this to me.

Roscam Abbing: I am glad that you made this comment. I am consciously a practicing Christian, but I do not think that I should speak from that point of view entirely. People who think differently also have the right to express their opinions. We must have general ethical notions which enable us to talk to one another on these points. Everyone's view of life is to be taken into consideration.

van de Vooren: I agree with Roscam Abbing that the registration of hereditary defects could be very useful. If, however, you introduce legislation for the obligatory registration of hereditary defects then the basic principles of medical ethics would be completely ignored.

Roscam Abbing: Central registration of such defects must be accessible to doctors or geneticists only. Information is already freely exchanged within the medical world, since that is in the interest of the patients. So it is really not a step further if you register genetic defects.

van de Vooren: I am afraid that if you use this registration to let the government decide that this child may be born and that child may not, families who come now to ask for advice will be frightened off.

Roscam Abbing: Yes, I recognize this problem, but I am not really in favour of the authorities stepping in; in the first instance, let us try to keep it on a voluntary basis. In the long run this may not be sufficient, so the authorities would have to intervene.

de Froe: We are now going to talk about abortion and its relationship, if any, to positive euthanasia.

Roscam Abbing: I should like eugenics to be as much part of the discussion as euthanasia and abortion. But abortion is indeed a question of prenatal positive euthanasia, active euthanasia. The question is whether abortion is justifiable, not only when we are sure from antenatal investigation that the foetus is affected, but also when we know that there is a 50% chance of a normal child. Usually, in The Netherlands, abortion under such circumstances would not raise many objections, but I still consider this a serious moral problem. But the problem is even worse if you delay the decision to break off life until after birth, although I do realize that no specific moment can be recognized as a cut off point or 'caesura'. The question is, why is 10 or 12 weeks or even 20 weeks accepted and not the moment of birth? In our culture birth is emotionally the most important moment, but in the final analysis I cannot see this as logical reasoning. And therefore, although with extreme hesitation, I can imagine that the life of a child born with a very severe mental defect could be cut off after birth. It seems to me that there is an essential difference as compared to an inherited disease manifesting itself well after birth.

In the latter case a relationship has been built between the parents and the child, it has been accepted; once accepted, one has to carry this acceptance right through.

de Froe: Perhaps Mr. Heering and Mr. Beemer can give their point of view on this subject.

Heering: I am glad that we are talking about abortion only in relation to the very defective child. In this context it seems to me that abortion has become a relatively simple problem. I of course agree with Roscam Abbing that life is a continuity, albeit in phases. You cannot say that birth is the definite 'caesura' and that no human life has existed before that, but this means that our ethics and actions must be interpreted in phases. I do not think that you can simply say that if we have accepted abortion we have also accepted euthanasia for newborn children. The most we can say is that euthanasia of newborn children is seen in a somewhat different light. Each phase demands its own decision. There is an important social aspect to this as well, which has not been brought up as yet.

Beemer: The value that people, society, assign to birth plays an important role in our argumentation. In talking about bearable and unbearable life, can we formulate our view of optimal life, and is it possible to set a limit below which life is unbearable? Can we agree on such maximums and minimums, and is it human to end a life that is below a minimum standard, thus defined?

Edwards: I think all this emphazises the extreme difficulty one encounters if one attempts to gain a little in one way by having a registry or by giving recommendations, since in another way one loses. We have it on the best authority that the good Shepherd follows one sheep and leaves ninety-nine to their faith, but in the practical world this does lead to difficulties, and this in particular I would like to mention in relation to maternal age. There does seem to be a very wide-spread belief that it is wrong for women to reproduce after the age of 30. There have been documents circulated in the United States, for example, saying that women over 35 should consult their physicians before conceiving. This is a problem, because mongolism is the only disease of any practical importance in which the frequency increases with maternal age. But there seems to be a strong positive maternal age effect in women above 30 who for economic reasons have an advantage over women under 30 in general. So what you lose in one respect by aging of the uterus or whatever it is that ages – the uterus may be at its peak in the twenties – you gain because the extra-uterine environment is in practice at its peak in the thirties; and if you are worried about childhood disease as a whole, rather than specifically worrying about mongolism which is not the major problem of any country, then I think one really must consider whether one should advise people to reproduce before 30 or after 30. Whatever you do in trying to change things for genetic benefits by discouraging reproduction above the age of 30, you in fact create another set of problems in forgetting that the best environment, on purely economic and social grounds, into which a child can be born tends to be that provided by women over 30.

Volker-Dieben: We have really only talked about dreadful suffering in connection with anencephaly and Down's syndrome. I want to give a practical example of a 25-year-old lawyer who is blind due to an X-linked condition. He knows that all his daughters would be carriers, and this makes him suffer so much that this man says: 'I will not have any daughters, even if they would be phenotypically normal.

I would not like them to suffer because they could have children who inherit this crippling disease'. Potential parents have a very important part to play in decision making, also in relation to selective abortion, when they are the ones who suffer.

Galjaard: I can agree with you. People who know from their own experience what suffering is and think that they can cope with that suffering are not the people who ask for prenatal advice. People who think that they might not be able to accept that pain and distress are the ones who do ask for prenatal examination. So we must leave room for the individual approach, unrestricted by legal measures concerning the maximum acceptable period for abortion.

de Froe: We shall have to come to a close. From the discussion this afternoon it is obvious that there are very different points of view regarding ethical questions in the prevention of inherited diseases. I hope that from these discussions we have been convinced that one should never feel self-satisfied and certain of having the only right answer. The possibility to review our opinions must always remain, and therefore discussion should never be closed.

INDEX OF SUBJECTS